Health Services Research:
Work Force and Educational Issues

Committee on Health Services Research: Training
and Work Force Issues

Marilyn J. Field, Robert E. Tranquada,
and Jill C. Feasley, *Editors*

Division of Health Care Services

INSTITUTE OF MEDICINE

NATIONAL ACADEMY PRESS
Washington, D.C. 1995

National Academy Press • 2101 Constitution Avenue, N.W. • Washington, D.C. 20418

NOTICE: The project that is the subject of this report was approved by the Governing Board of the National Research Council, whose members are drawn from the councils of the National Academy of Sciences, the National Academy of Engineering, and the Institute of Medicine. The members of the committee responsible for the report were chosen for their special competences and with regard for appropriate balance.

This report has been reviewed by a group other than the authors according to procedures approved by a Report Review Committee consisting of members of the National Academy of Sciences, the National Academy of Engineering, and the Institute of Medicine.

The Institute of Medicine was chartered in 1970 by the National Academy of Sciences to enlist distinguished members of the appropriate professions in the examination of policy matters pertaining to the health of the public. In this, the Institute acts under both the Academy's 1863 congressional charter responsibility to be an adviser to the federal government and its own initiative in identifying issues of medical care, research, and education. Dr. Kenneth I. Shine is president of the Institute of Medicine.

Support for this project was provided by the Agency for Health Care Policy and Research, U.S. Department of Health and Human Services, under Contract No. 282-94-2008; the Robert Wood Johnson Foundation, under Grant No. 24791; the Department of Veterans Affairs; and the Baxter Foundation. The views presented are those of the Institute of Medicine Committee on Health Services Research Training and Work Force Issues and are not necessarily those of the funding organizations.

Library of Congress Catalog Card No. 95-71398
International Standard Book No. 0-309-05348-X

Additional copies of this report are available from:

National Academy Press
2101 Constitution Avenue, N.W.
Box 285
Washington, D.C. 20055
Call 800-624-6242 (or 202-334-3313 in the Washington metropolitan area)

The serpent has been a symbol of long life, healing, and knowledge among almost all cultures and religions since the beginning of recorded history. The image adopted as a logotype by the Institute of Medicine is based on a relief carving from ancient Greece, now held by the Staatlichemuseen in Berlin.

Printed in the United States of America

COMMITTEE ON HEALTH SERVICES RESEARCH: TRAINING AND WORK FORCE ISSUES

ROBERT E. TRANQUADA,* *Chair,* Norman Topping/National Medical Enterprises Professor of Medicine and Public Policy, University of Southern California, Los Angeles, California

PAULA K. DIEHR, Professor, Department of Biostatistics, University of Washington, Seattle, Washington

DEBORAH A. FREUND, Vice Chancellor, Academic Affairs, and Dean of Faculties, Indiana University, Bloomington, Indiana

WILLIAM T. FRIEDEWALD, Senior Vice President and Chief Medical Director, Metropolitan Life Insurance Company, New York, New York (resigned January 17, 1995)

JOHN C. GREENE,* Professor and Dean Emeritus, School of Dentistry, University of California, San Francisco, California

MERWYN R. GREENLICK,* Professor and Chair, Department of Public Health and Preventive Medicine, Oregon Health Sciences University, and Director, Kaiser Permanente Center for Health Research, Portland, Oregon

ADA SUE HINSHAW,* Dean, School of Nursing, University of Michigan, Ann Arbor, Michigan

DAVID A. KINDIG, Professor of Preventive Medicine, and Director, Wisconsin Network for Health Policy Research, University of Wisconsin–Madison School of Medicine, Madison, Wisconsin

KENNETH W. KIZER, Professor and Chair, Departments of Community and International Health, School of Medicine, University of California, Davis, California (position at time of committee service, resigned October 24, 1994)

KEVIN J. LYONS, Associate Dean and Director, Center for Collaborative Research, College of Allied Health Sciences, Thomas Jefferson University, Philadelphia, Pennsylvania

ALBERT G. MULLEY, Chief, General Internal Medicine Unit, Massachusetts General Hospital, Boston, Massachusetts

WILLIAM L. ROPER,* Senior Vice President and Chief Medical Officer, The Prudential Health Care System, Atlanta, Georgia

DONALD M. STEINWACHS,* Chair and Professor, Department of Health Policy and Management, Johns Hopkins University School of Hygiene and Public Health, Baltimore, Maryland

BAILUS WALKER, Jr.,* Professor of Environmental and Occupational Medicine, and Associate Director, University Cancer Center, Howard University College of Medicine, Washington, D.C.

---

* Member, Institute of Medicine

Study Staff

MARILYN J. FIELD, Study Director (after January 15, 1995)
JILL C. FEASLEY, Research Associate (after October 1, 1994)
DONNA D. THOMPSON, Administrative Assistant (through May 5, 1995)
KATHLEEN N. LOHR, Director, Division of Health Care Services
SUSAN THAUL, Study Director (through January 15, 1995)
KARLA R. SAUNDERS, Administrative Assistant (after June 12, 1995)
NINA H. SPRUILL, Financial Officer

Acknowledgments

The Committee on Health Services Research: Training and Work Force Issues wants to acknowledge those who assisted it in preparing this report. At the Agency for Health Care Policy and Research, James Cooper, the project officer, helped us in many ways. Donnarae Castillo, who is responsible for the National Research Service Award activities within the agency, patiently answered questions and compiled information on institutional and individual awards. Ralph Sloat helped us locate difficult-to-find historical information about earlier training activities. Julius Rosenthal at the Agency for Health Care Policy Research supplied information on dissertation research awards. At the Department of Veterans Affairs (VA), Shirley Meehan and Joseph Gouch provided information on the Health Services Research educational programs at the VA.

Within the National Research Council, Porter Coggeshall, Pamela Ebert-Flattau, Anthony DeSantis, and others provided information about the series of studies of biomedical and behavioral science research personnel that the Office of Scientific and Engineering Personnel has conducted since 1975.

With support from the Pew Health Policy Program, Marion Lewin and Valerie Tate Jopeck, colleagues within the Institute of Medicine (IOM), contributed substantially to committee efforts to gain perspectives from private industry and state government. They helped organize a panel of industry representatives for the committee's March 1995 meeting in which the committee heard from Howard Bailit, Henry Bachofer, Carmela Dyer, Lawrence Lewin, and Bruce Steinwald. Marion Lewin also participated in telephone interviews with current and former state officials including Mark Chassin, Dennis Beatrice, Robert Crittenden, Robert Frank, Alan Weil, Pamela Paul-Sheehan, Beth Kilbreth, and Richard Merritt. The committee also expresses its appreciation to the two dozen executives of health plans, consulting firms, and similar organizations who agreed to be interviewed by committee members about health services researchers in private industry.

At the University of Wisconsin–Madison, Nancy Cross Dunham and Karen Tyler of the Wisconsin Network for Health Policy Research created the health services researcher database for the committee and drafted a report describing the method and results. That database is more comprehensive than any developed before. Alice Hersh, Suzan Meredith, and Jennifer Rotchford of the Association for Health Services Research provided considerable information including their membership files.

As usual, staff at the IOM provided critical support for the work of the committee and project staff. They include Elizabeth Mouzon, Donna Thompson, Don Tiller, Nina Spruill, Susan Thaul, Dorothy Majewski, Sarah Reich, Claudia Carl, Mike Edington, and Richard Julian. An especially heartfelt thank-you goes to Mary Lee Schneiders who spent many long hours working through the complexities of database conversion and manipulation.

Contents

TABLES AND FIGURES

TABLES

FIGURES

Health Services Research:
Work Force and Educational Issues

Summary

Health services research is a multidisciplinary field that investigates the structure, processes, and effects of health care services. It draws on a variety of clinical and academic disciplines and, at its most creative, integrates their conceptual frameworks and methods to provide new ways of studying and understanding the health care system.

This system is the product of scientific, technological, and social developments that have dramatically expanded the capabilities of medical care during the past century. Health services research and education were born of demands for better information and analysis to guide complex decisions about the organization, financing, and effectiveness of health care.

Recently, the health care system has been experiencing a dramatic restructuring. Governments and employers have intensified their efforts to direct people into managed care plans that control patient access to practitioners and services, pay providers fixed amounts for a defined set of services to a defined set of patients, and otherwise manage the use and cost of care. Health care organizations are consolidating, expanding, shrinking, reorganizing, or otherwise changing in ways that are varied, sometimes perplexing, and unclear in their effects on the cost, quality, and accessibility of health care. In this environment of rapid change and uncertainty, health services research has an important contribution to make in documenting and evaluating the effects of health care restructuring. Furthermore, just as health services research has helped decisionmakers understand and shape the health care system of the past, so too can it continue to inform critical decisions by government officials, corporate leaders, clinicians, health plan managers, and even ordinary people making choices about health problems ranging from minor to catastrophic.

The federal government is the major sponsor as well as an important consumer of health services research. Funding for health services research and education has, however, been decreasing as a share of total health spending, comprising a smaller percentage of total health spending in 1990 than in 1970. As this report was being completed, the drive to balance the federal budget was intensifying pressures on this funding and threatening the existence of the lead federal agency for health services research. Private organizations, including foundations and managed care plans, can be expected to continue and possibly increase their investment in some areas of health services research. Nonetheless, foundations are facing heavy pressure to use their resources to offset some reductions in public spending for social programs. Among health care organizations, intense price competition limits resources for research that does not promise a short-term competitive advantage. Taken as a whole, private efforts are unlikely to substitute for more than a portion of government-supported research and training in magnitude, coherence, scope, or concern for long-term consequences. In this environment, sustaining the capacity for high-quality health services research and training will be a formidable task.

ORIGINS OF THE STUDY

This report focuses on one part of the field of health services research—its work force and its programs for educating and training that work force. The study originated in a request from the Agency for Health Care Policy and Research (AHCPR), which was created by Congress in 1989 to support research, data development, and other activities that will "enhance the quality, appropriateness, and effectiveness of health care services" (P.L. 101-239). Other support was provided by the Robert Wood Johnson Foundation, the Department of Veterans Affairs, and the Baxter Foundation.

AHCPR asked the Institute of Medicine (IOM) to investigate work force issues in health services research and prepare a report with recommendations to inform the agency's decisions about federal resources for educating and training health services researchers. Among the questions posed to the committee were: (1) What health services research personnel and training resources are available now? (2) What levels and types of personnel may be needed in the next decade? (3) What changes in programs and resources may be necessary to meet future demand for health services researchers? The IOM was not asked to evaluate the content of the nation's research agenda, the adequacy of overall research funding, or the productivity of research activities, although these issues are clearly worthy of examination in their own right.

STUDY APPROACH

To oversee the study, the IOM appointed a 12-member committee. It included individuals with expertise and experience in health services research, research training, health care delivery, public policy, and economics. The committee met in July 1994, January 1995, and March 1995. After discovering the paucity of current and trend data on the size and characteristics of the health services research work force, the committee obtained private funding to undertake quickly a number of information collection activities, including

- a survey of directors of health services research training programs in the United States and Canada;
- creation of a database of health services researchers in the United States; and
- telephone interviews or panel discussions with key individuals in state governments, managed care organizations, hospital systems, consulting firms, and other nonacademic organizations.

The committee also consulted two related studies by other units within the National Academy complex. One, *Meeting the Nation's Needs for Biomedical and Behavioral Scientists* (NRC, 1994), was the latest in a series of National Research Council (NRC) reports on this topic, and the other, *Reshaping the Graduate Education of Scientists and Engineers* (1995), focused broadly on challenges for graduate education in science and engineering.

In September 1994, the committee published an interim statement that included a working definition of health services research and a review of important research questions. Responses to that statement contributed to the development of the committee's final report, which was reviewed and revised under the procedures of the NRC.

DEFINING HEALTH SERVICES RESEARCH

After reviewing various definitions of health services research, the committee formulated the following definition:

Health services research is a multidisciplinary field of inquiry, both basic and applied, that examines the use, costs, quality, accessibility, delivery, organization, financing, and outcomes of health care services to increase knowledge and understanding of the structure, processes, and effects of health services for individuals and populations.

Several features of this definition are worth noting. First, health services research is a *multidisciplinary field* that draws from many distinct academic and clinical disciplines such as economics, epidemiology, biostatistics, and nursing. This characteristic of the field complicates efforts to catalog and analyze its processes, participants, and products.

Second, the definition's reference to *basic and applied* research underscores the fact that health service research involves both questions about fundamental individual and institutional behaviors that may not produce practically useful knowledge in the short term, as well as questions of immediate practical interest to public and private decisionmakers. In general, health services research falls toward the applied end of the research continuum.

Third, by referring to both *knowledge* and *understanding,* the definition stretches the boundaries of the field to include not only research that generates new knowledge but also analyses that contribute to the theoretical and conceptual frameworks for conducting, interpreting, and applying empirical research. Thus, the boundaries of health services research, health care management, and health policy are not sharp.

Finally, this definition does not explicitly restrict research to personal health services. Rather, it makes clear that the health of *populations*—as well as that of *individuals*—is a relevant research topic. As more individuals are enrolled in managed care plans, interest has grown in measuring and comparing quality and cost performance at the group level and in assessing the relative contribution of clinical interventions to the well-being of the group as well as that of its individual members.

This report uses the terms *education* and *training* interchangeably, as is common in the health professions. Conceptually, however, education may be viewed as transmitting broad knowledge relevant to a field and developing critical thinking abilities that are widely viewed as essential to the creation and evaluation of new knowledge. Training may be more narrowly defined as providing the skills (e.g., facility in statistics and survey design) that are necessary for specific research activities (e.g., preparing surveys, analyzing data).

FINDINGS AND RECOMMENDATIONS

Work Force Data

One of the committee's first findings was that existing data on the size and characteristics of the health services research work force are fragmentary and incomplete. The committee urges

• the Association for Health Services Research (AHSR) to seek funding to update and extend the database created for this study through a more detailed survey of researcher characteristics including, for example, age, sex, ethnicity, and employment status;

• the NRC to consider revising the annual census of those who have received doctorates and the longitudinal sample survey of doctoral recipients to allow better identification of those educated or working in the field of health services research;

• the AHCPR and other relevant government agencies—as part of a more general effort to evaluate the results of various research training programs—to investigate the career paths and productivity of those who receive trainee grants or fellowship awards.

These recommendations are consistent with those of the 1995 NRC report *Reshaping the Graduate Education of Scientists and Engineers.* That report urged the National Science Foundation and the NRC to continue to improve the coverage, timeliness, and analysis of education and employment data to support more informed decisions about the country's science and technology work force. A more specific recommendation was that additional information on nonacademic employment be gathered, given the growing importance of this sector.

Work Force Supply and Demand

The work force engaged in health services research has three broad components: (1) researchers who originate, design, supervise, and report basic and applied health services research; (2) individuals who assist in health services research under the direction of others; and (3) individuals who analyze health services information and apply certain tools of health services research in management and policy settings. The boundaries of the health services research work force (and its individual components) are, however, highly permeable. People come to the field by many paths, some through formal education and others through relevant work experience. Similarly, those trained in health services research may migrate to work that uses their skills but is quite different from traditional academic or think tank employment. This permeability adds to the problems in counting the research work force. These problems are accentuated to the extent that some researchers choose to identify themselves with their primary discipline (e.g., economics or medicine) rather than with health services research.

Using its multiple databases, the committee identified approximately 5,000 current health services researchers. As an estimate of the size of the work force, this number omits some health services researchers and includes some individuals who are interested in health services research but not actually engaged in it. Approximately half of the researchers for whom degree information was available have doctoral degrees, but the specific field or discipline could not be determined, and another 28 percent (mostly physicians) have clinical degrees.

The largest segments of the current health services research work force appear to be employed in academic institutions, private research organizations, and consulting groups. Employment in health plans, insurance companies, and similar organizations appears to be growing fast, albeit from a smaller base. The picture for states, which generally contract out for research rather than maintain research staff, suggests severe financial pressure on research projects except for those related to costly programs such as Medicaid. For graduate scientists and engineers in general, academic jobs are declining while positions in business and industry are growing.

Without information on researchers' age, employment history, or percentage of time spent in research, life table models or other work force estimation methods cannot be employed to arrive at reasonable numerical projections of the future supply of health services researchers. On qualitative grounds, however, the committee foresees expansion in the health services research work force *if* public research funding escapes significant reductions and *if* organizations competing in the emerging health care market continue to support growth in knowledge about the quality, effectiveness, and cost of clinical services, the behavioral determinants of health status, and similar questions.

The committee also was not able to make an empirically based, quantitative statement about the match between current supply and current demand for health services researchers. Based on limited information from health services research employers and on the experience of committee members, the committee concluded that well-trained researchers with practical experience in health care organizations (e.g., integrated health care systems, insurance companies) and in managing research units appear to be in short supply. In addition, recruiting difficulties were reported for those trained in both health services research and selected areas, including outcomes and health status measurement, epidemiology, health economics, statistics, epidemiology, and health policy. In some clinical areas, such as oral health and allied health services, trained health services researchers also appear to be scarce.

Overall, the committee reached two qualitative conclusions. First, no anecdotal or other evidence indicates that the current supply of health services researchers exceeds current demand. Second, employers are more concerned about the quality than the quantity of prospective researchers.

Training Programs

Funding for education in health services research comes from a variety of public and private sources. With funds provided by the National Institutes of Health under general authority of the National Research Service Award (NRSA) Act, AHCPR administers the major federal funding program for pre- and postdoctoral education in health services research. The program, which AHCPR has also supplemented through its own budget, provides awards both to institutions and to individuals.

Health services research education and training are provided under many different organizational auspices, for example, as part of doctoral programs in health policy and administration, public health, nursing, social work, biostatistics, and economics. The committee noted, however, that formal programs in health services research play a special role by providing an organizing focus for the field and an environment supportive of creative research and methodology development. They stimulate systematic, multidisciplinary investigation and understanding of health services, behaviors, and outcomes, and they promote the formulation of research frameworks and strategies that integrate the theories, concepts, and tools of different disciplines. These programs are also an important source of personnel prepared to increase the knowledge base for responding to issues of cost, quality, and access that face the nation. They are, therefore, a valuable national resource.

A single educational path is, however, neither practical nor desirable. Health services research will continue to attract and benefit from people with a variety of disciplinary and clinical degrees who are prepared to make important theoretical, conceptual, and empirical contributions to the field. To take full advantage of this variety, the field needs to offer a range of training opportunities so that those who are pursuing or have completed graduate degrees in other areas can obtain explicit training in health services research through either a disciplinary or, ideally, a multidisciplinary program.

As this study proceeded, the committee became concerned that those in doctoral programs were not being adequately prepared for the "real world" (or worlds) of health services research. Given the nature of the field, researchers will often find themselves working as part of a research team with individuals from varied disciplinary or clinical backgrounds and different levels of training and experience. The committee was concerned that students are not routinely educated to understand what may reasonably be expected from other researchers or clinicians, to value the contributions of master's-level researchers, or to develop the qualities needed to lead or participate effectively in a research team. Such qualities include communication skills, facility in group decisionmaking processes, and knowledge of conflict resolution strategies. Given recent trends in employment, it is the general sense of the committee that health services research programs will benefit their students by providing broad educational opportunities that make them more versatile, flexible, and attractive to corporate and governmental as well as academic employers. These opportunities include course work in several disciplines and methodological techniques, practical experience in research and policy analysis, and exposure to differences in expectations for researchers among academic, government, and industry employers. Academic programs cannot substitute for on-the-job education, but they can make entry to a new work setting somewhat easier.

Based on changing sources and types of demand for health services researchers, some shifts in the focus of publicly supported training in health services research are advisable. In particular, the committee recommended that AHCPR

• consider greater emphasis for some predoctoral and postdoctoral awards for training in areas such as outcomes/health status measurement, biostatistics, epidemiology, health economics, and health policy in which recruiting difficulties have been reported;

• more explicitly consider—in evaluating institutional training program awards—how institutions' approaches to training, faculty composition, research opportunities, and training slots relate to high-demand areas; and

• set aside a substantial percentage of institutional awards for innovative programs in health services research, which could be completely new programs or significant modifications of existing programs (see below).

The committee offered no ranked prescription for the program innovations to be encouraged. By way of example, however, innovative programs might be designed to

• explore new models and methods for truly multidisciplinary education and investigation;

• test creative educational opportunities and technologies for mid career professionals who have varied levels and kinds of educational backgrounds and work experiences;

• extend student and faculty research experiences in nonacademic settings through mechanisms such as internships and faculty sabbaticals;

• develop strategies to involve more community-based practitioners in faculty research on clinical practice and its outcomes; or

• cultivate partnerships with public or private organizations to encourage collaborative research training, joint methodology development, and other cooperative ventures.

Several of these examples point toward programs that are more community and customer oriented; that is, programs that better prepare students for employment in government, business, and academic settings. Such innovative steps may be somewhat more costly than current programs and may require additional public and private support.

The committee also reviewed and endorsed the recommendations for health services research training awards that were issued in the 1994 NRC report *Meeting the Nation's Needs on Biomedical and Behavioral Scientists.* The recommendations called for

- funding 360 NRSA yearly for fiscal years 1996 through 1999;
- raising stipends to more competitive levels by fiscal year 1996 and maintaining the real value of these stipends by adjusting for inflation;
- examining research training opportunities for women through the NRSA program and strengthening the role of postdoctoral support to assist women in establishing themselves in productive research careers; and
- holding Minority Access to Research Careers awards constant at fiscal 1993 levels, or approximately 680 awards, pending the outcome of further analyses.

HEALTH SERVICES RESEARCH: TODAY AND TOMORROW

Health service researchers face no shortage of important, contentious questions and methodologic challenges. Among the critical areas for continued attention are the following:

Organization and financing of health services. Health services research can inform the debate over incremental reforms in health insurance and market-based strategies to control health care costs. It can, for example, clarify the complexities of maintaining and overseeing health insurance markets, in particular, the peculiar dilemmas presented by adverse risk selection and the difficulties of devising methods for paying health plans and providers and monitoring their performance so that they are discouraged from avoiding sicker people or skimping on the quality of care.

Access to health care. Research continues to document how access—the timely receipt of appropriate care—is affected by insurance coverage, levels of payment to providers of care, race, culture, and other factors and how, in turn, lack of access affects health. Continued work in these areas is important for informed policy choices.

Practitioner, patient, and consumer behavior. Although researchers have identified many factors affecting health behavior, much remains to be learned about ways of encouraging desired behaviors, such as cost-effective use of medical care and compliance with preventive or treatment protocols.

Quality of care. Health services research has played and will continue to play a critical role in developing and improving mechanisms for identifying quality of care problems and measuring the performance of health plans and clinicians in a competitive market. One priority (a corollary of the point above about adverse selection) is the development of better methods of adjusting comparative data so that the performance of those who treat sicker patients is fairly rated.

Clinical evaluation and outcomes research. A major recent emphasis in health services research has been clinical evaluative studies and outcomes research on the benefits and harms of alternative strategies for preventing, diagnosing, or treating illness. Work to date only scratches the surface of ignorance about what works and does not work in health care.

Informatics and clinical decisionmaking. Health services researchers have found serious deficits in the ways in which knowledge is packaged and disseminated to inform decisionmakers. A major goal of information systems technologies is to help patients, clinicians, purchasers, and policymakers make better decisions about health care.

Health professions work force. As this committee confirmed, efforts to forecast, plan, and manage the supply of health personnel and services have proved difficult. Methodologists and researchers are working to improve data systems and tools for estimating work force supply and demand.

In each of these areas, health services researchers investigate important and fascinating issues that profoundly affect the health and well-being of individuals and populations. They develop and apply methodologies and analytic frameworks to understand the structure, processes, and effects of health care services and provide a more informed basis for decisions by public officials, clinicians, patients, health plan managers, and others.

This report has examined a critical component of the health services research enterprise—its work force and its programs for educating and training that work force. The conclusions reflect the committee's judgment that this work force plays an important role in providing information and tools that are necessary for an effectively functioning health care market and an accountable health care system. Its contributions will become even more significant for patients, clinicians, managers, and policymakers as the effects of unprecedented changes in health care delivery and financing are more widely experienced. These contributions are unlikely to be sustained by private efforts if public funding is significantly reduced. Like research and education in the biomedical and clinical sciences, generally, health services research and research training are public goods worthy of support by society as a whole.

1

Introduction and Background

When faced with the same symptoms, why do some people seek medical care and others avoid contact with health care providers?

*

How do different instruments for measuring patient health status compare in their ability to adjust data on health plan costs, services, or health outcomes to control for differences in the health status of plan members?

*

How do capitated, per case, or other methods for paying health care institutions and practitioners affect the provision of appropriate and inappropriate medical services and the outcomes of care?

*

What kinds of preventive, therapeutic, or other services can be safely and effectively provided by health professionals such as physical therapists, dental hygienists, and other allied health providers?

*

What are the strengths and weaknesses of current federal approaches to the regulation of pharmaceuticals and devices in making beneficial products available to patients?

*

Is the growth of managed care affecting clinical research and technological innovation?

Health services researchers investigate questions such as these. The answers that researchers provide can guide critical decisions by government officials, corporate leaders, clinicians, health plan managers, and ordinary people experiencing health problems ranging from minor to life threatening. Unfortunately, many important decisions closely connected to these and similar questions must now be made in the absence of adequate knowledge of the likely consequences of different choices. The challenge for health services research is to reduce this knowledge gap.

This report focuses on one part of the health services research enterprise—its work force and its programs for educating and training that work force. The rest of this chapter reviews the origins of the study, describes the study strategy, and defines key terms. Chapter 2 discusses the evolution of health services research, presents major themes and questions addressed by current research, and considers how emphases may shift in the future. Chapter 3 examines the size and characteristics of the current health services research work force, the match between supply and demand for this work force, and issues in estimating work force requirements for the future. Chapter 4 focuses on health services research education and training programs. In Chapter 5, the committee presents its findings and recommendations. The Institute of Medicine (IOM) was not asked to evaluate the content of the nation's research agenda, the adequacy of overall research funding, or the productivity of research activities, although these issues are clearly worthy of examination.

ORIGINS OF THE STUDY

This study originated in a request from the Agency for Health Care Policy and Research (AHCPR), a unit of the U.S. Department of Health and Human Services. AHCPR was created by Congress in 1989 to support research, data development, and other activities that will "enhance the quality, appropriateness, and effectiveness of health care services" (P.L. 101-239). The legislation reflected policymakers' interest in acquiring a better knowledge base for guiding public and private decisions about health and health care. AHCPR is the largest single funder of health services research and health services research education in this country, although the various institutes of the National Institutes of Health, taken together, spend more. Other government agencies, private foundations, insurers, managed care plans, and additional organizations also sponsor research and, to a lesser extent, research education and training.

AHCPR asked the IOM to investigate work force issues in health services research and prepare a report with recommendations to inform decisions about federal resources for educating and training health services researchers. Among the questions posed were: What levels and types of trained health services research personnel are available now? What personnel may be needed in the next decade? What changes in programs and resources may be necessary to meet future demand for health services researchers?

When the study was first discussed, many policymakers anticipated that health reform legislation would be enacted at the federal level and that such reform would generate more questions for health services research and more resources (including education and training funds) for investigation. That reform did not materialize, and significant federal action appears unlikely for the immediate future. Research resources may actually be cut as part of initiatives to reduce the budget deficit or cut federal taxes.

Federal inaction notwithstanding, a restructuring of the health care delivery system—driven primarily by cost concerns and by the independent actions of a great many private organizations—is proceeding with surprising speed. Although economic considerations have been the immediate determinants of change, past research on the organization, financing, use, and outcomes of health care has influenced the direction of these changes in some measure, particularly in areas involving financial incentives, data reporting and analysis, and evaluation of treatment options and patterns. Regardless of its antecedents, health care restructuring raises significant questions and presents information-gathering challenges for the field of health services research and its supporting education and training programs.

STUDY APPROACH

To oversee the study, the IOM appointed a 12-member committee. It included individuals with expertise and experience in health services research, research training, health care delivery, public policy, and economics (see Appendix D).

The committee met in July 1994, January 1995, and March 1995. It undertook a number of information collection activities. Because health services research lacks licensure or certification processes to aid in the identification and enumeration of health services researchers, the committee used a "building block" strategy that combined several components to develop a database of health services researchers in the United States (see Chapter 3 and Appendix A). In addition, IOM staff surveyed directors of health services research training programs in the United States and Canada about various matters, including recent applications for admission, acceptance rates, students' academic and work experience, financial aid, curriculum, and employment of program graduates (see Chapter 4 and Appendix B).[1]

To investigate the interests of private industry and state government in health services research, committee members and staff conducted telephone interviews with more than two dozen key individuals in managed care organizations, hospital systems, consulting firms, state agencies, and other organizations. In addition, a panel of executives and researchers from these organizations met with the committee during its March 1995 meeting to discuss the focus of public and private sector research, policies on peer review and dissemination, and implications for health services research education and training.

The committee found the literature on educational and work force policies in the field of health services research to be sparse. Much of it appears in a series of reports on personnel needs and training for biomedical and behavioral research prepared by the National Research Council (NRC) and the IOM (NRC, 1975a, b, 1976, 1977, 1978, 1981, 1994; IOM, 1983, 1985). The most recent report (from the NRC's Office of Scientific and Engineering Personnel), *Meeting the Nation's Needs for Biomedical and Behavioral Scientists*, reviewed models for estimating supply and need for these personnel and made recommendations in several areas, including health services research (NRC, 1994). In addition, the committee consulted *Reshaping the Graduate Education of Scientists and Engineers,* a report of the Academy's Commission on Science, Engineering, and Public Policy (COSEPUP, 1995). The current IOM committee also reviewed the 1979 IOM report *Health Services Research* but determined that it did not investigate work force and training issues in any depth.

In September 1994, the committee published an interim statement that included a working definition of health services research and a review of important research questions (IOM, 1994a). Responses to that statement contributed to the development of the committee's final report, which was reviewed under the procedures of the NRC.

---

[1]Because government policies limit contractors' use of certain information collection strategies, the training program survey, the creation of the researcher database, and a series of telephone interviews with state and private officials were made possible by grants from the Robert Wood Johnson Foundation and the Baxter Foundation and by support from the Pew Health Policy Program at the IOM.

DEFINITIONS AND CONCEPTS

Health Services Research

The 1979 IOM report on health services research defined the field as "inquiry to produce knowledge about the structure, processes, or effects of personal health services" (p. 14). A study would be classified as health services research if it satisfied two criteria: (1) "it deals with some features of the structure, processes, or effects of personal health services" and (2) "at least one of the features is related to a conceptual framework other than that of contemporary applied biomedical science" (p. 14). It is implicit that such research could investigate the effects of personal health services on the health of populations but its primary focus would not be public health interventions (e.g., community-wide water fluoridation or education programs) as such.

A 1991 IOM report on information services for health services research, which was prepared for the National Library of Medicine, catalogued various definitions of health services research dating back 20 years (IOM, 1991). That study committee did not formally adopt the 1979 definition or develop a definition of its own but noted common features of many definitions, including a focus on populations as well as individuals.

The current committee also consulted other definitions and descriptions (e.g., Flook and Sanazaro, 1973; Steinwachs, 1991). Building on these earlier statements, the committee formulated the following definition:

> Health services research is a multidisciplinary field of inquiry, both basic and applied, that examines the use, costs, quality, accessibility, delivery, organization, financing, and outcomes of health care services to increase knowledge and understanding of the structure, processes, and effects of health services for individuals and populations.

Several features of this definition are worth noting. First, health services research is a *multidisciplinary field* that draws from many distinct academic and clinical disciplines such as economics, epidemiology, biostatistics, and nursing.[2] Its boundaries are imprecise, particularly as they relate to policy and management

---

[2] Although it recognized that the terms are often used interchangeably and are not clearly differentiated by dictionaries, the committee concluded that a distinction between *multidisciplinary* and *interdisciplinary* would be useful. It suggests that the first term generally be used to describe work that *involves* multiple disciplines and that the second term be reserved for work that attempts to *integrate* disciplines in ways that forge new frameworks and strategies for investigation.

studies and certain kinds of clinical research.[3] Specific instances of research may exemplify the multidisciplinary aspect of the field to varying degrees. For example, an epidemiologist studying the effects of a particular vaccination program on the incidence of a particular disease might or might not consider social, economic, organizational, or similar factors affecting (or affected by) the rate or distribution of vaccinations. Absent such consideration, the research would not fit the definition of health services research offered here (unless, perhaps, it were undertaken in conjunction with a broader project).

Second, the definition's reference to *basic and applied* research underscores the fact that health service research involves both questions about fundamental individual, organization, and system behaviors and questions of direct practical interest to public and private decisionmakers. In general, health services research falls toward the applied end of the research continuum. Many university-based health services research and training programs are located in or described as health management and policy programs, clearly emphasizing their concern with applications. Applied research, particularly that involving the effectiveness of medical interventions and the use (or nonuse) of the resulting information by patients and practitioners, is the major focus of work funded by AHCPR. With support from both public and private sources, health services researchers have devised better measures of health status and the severity of illnesses. They have also contributed to the development of methods for paying for hospital care and physician services that reduce financial incentives for the overuse of inpatient care, medical procedures, and specialty services. Researchers are now intensifying their efforts to develop tools to detect underuse of appropriate care and to adjust provider payments in ways that discourage providers from skimping on care or avoiding high-risk individuals.

Third, by referring to both *knowledge* and *understanding,* the definition stretches the boundaries of the field to include not only research that generates new knowledge but also analyses that contribute to the theoretical and conceptual frameworks for conducting, interpreting, and applying empirical research. For example, Donabedian's influential writings on quality assessment and assurance would fall in the latter category (Donabedian, 1966, 1980, 1982, 1985).

---

[3]The ADAMHA Reorganization Act of 1992 (42 USC § 284d) defined health services research as "research endeavors that study the impact of the organization, financing and management of health services on the quality, cost, access to and outcomes of care. Such term does not include research on the efficacy of services to prevent, diagnose, or treat medical conditions." The committee assumes that the latter exclusion refers to clinical research, in particular, controlled clinical trials rather than research in real-world settings (see Brook and Lohr, 1985, for a discussion of the difference between efficacy and effectiveness). Depending on its design, a clinical trial would not necessarily be excluded under the committee's definition.

Finally, compared to the 1979 definition of health services research, the one offered here does not explicitly restrict research to personal health services. Rather, it makes clear that the health of *populations* as well as that of *individuals* is a relevant research topic. As more individuals are enrolled in managed care plans, interest has grown in measuring and comparing quality and cost performance at the group level and in assessing the relative contribution of clinical interventions to the well-being of the group as well as that of its individual members.

Investigators can define populations in many different ways based on sociodemographic characteristics, geographic location, or enrollment in different health insurance plans. Traditionally, population-based health services have been conceived of in terms of community-wide health education programs, surveillance activities, communicable disease control methods, and similar programs. Now, large health care delivery organizations are managing personal health services for an increasing proportion of the population, and more efforts are being made to define organizational policies with a view to their effects on their defined populations rather than given individuals. These developments present health services researchers with important questions about how organizational structures and processes affect the health and well-being of subject populations.

Health Services Research Work Force

Just as delineating the scope of health services research is not a straightforward task, neither is identifying the health services research work force. In contrast to the clinical health professions that have licensure and specific degree requirements as key defining characteristics, one is not required to have a license or a specific degree to practice health services research—or most other kinds of research, for that matter. Unlike health services researchers, however, those in biomedical and behavioral research fields generally can be identified by specific disciplines (e.g., biochemistry, psychology) and counted as such in periodic surveys of individuals who have earned or are working toward doctorates (NRC, 1994).

The committee distinguished three broad components of the health services research work force. As depicted in Figure 1.1, they include

• investigators who originate, design, supervise, and report basic and applied health services research;
• researchers who assist in health services research under the direction of others; and

• individuals who analyze health services information and apply certain tools of health services research in management and policy settings.

In general, the first category requires preparation at the doctoral level or equivalent, whereas the latter two categories usually require master's-level or other advanced training. Depending on their preparation and role, clinicians may be found in any of the three categories. As noted earlier, it is difficult to distinguish the health services research field from the arenas of clinical research, health care management, and health policymaking.

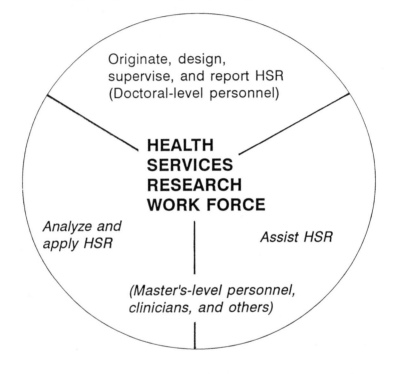

FIGURE 1.1 U.S. health services research (HSR) work force, by function. Please note that the boundaries are not precise.

Health Services Research Education and Training

This report uses the terms *education* and *training* interchangeably, as is common in the health professions. Conceptually, however, *education* may be viewed as transmitting broad knowledge relevant to a field and developing critical thinking abilities that are widely viewed as essential to the creation and evaluation of new knowledge. Training may be more narrowly defined as providing the skills (e.g., facility in statistics and survey design) that are necessary for specific research activities (e.g., preparing surveys, analyzing data, reporting results).

Education and training for health services research can occur in many settings ranging from universities to government institutes and private seminars. Although the committee attempted to learn more about nonuniversity settings, it emphasized academic programs in part because of data availability and in part because federal training funds are largely focused on such institutions and their students.

Education and training opportunities also vary by level or intensity. This report considers three categories: (1) predoctoral education that leads to a research doctorate in health services research or a relevant discipline; (2) post-doctoral education that provides formal, specialized training and research experience for those with research or clinical doctorates; and (3) master's-level education that prepares individuals to participate in research. In addition, the report notes that continuing education is an important resource, both to inform new or established researchers about advances in knowledge or methods and to assist people in shifting career paths as employment opportunities contract or expand in different sectors.

Support for Health Services Research

As is also the case for biomedical and clinical research, the federal government clearly is the major sponsor of health services research and research training. Although the lead governmental agency for health services research is nominally AHCPR, other agencies also fund significant amounts of research (see Table 1.1).

Some research areas—in particular, technology assessment, quality assessment including outcomes research, and data systems—are also attracting industry funding, generally for work that will support corporate objectives and decisionmaking needs. For example, researchers with an understanding of pharmacoeconomics are in high demand from drug companies attempting to nfluence or respond to market and regulatory shifts and uncertainties. State governments also support some health services research, primarily through contracts with outside organizations. The committee did not find specific information about the aggregate level and distribution of health services research funding provided by private foundations, corporations, state governments, and other sources.

TABLE 1.1 Federal Expenditures for Health Services Research, FY 1994 and 1995 Appropriations (in millions of dollars)

Agency[a]	FY 1994	FY 1995
AHCPR	152	160[b]
NIMH	92	95
NIDA	64	66
NIAAA	28	29
NLM	8	8
HCFA/ORD	43	46
VA/HSR&D	31	32
TOTAL	418	436

NOTE: Other institutes fund health services research but do not identify it as such. The National Cancer Institute; the National Heart, Blood, and Lung Institute; and the National Institute on Aging all have significant research activities concerned with the provision of services and the effectiveness of care within their categorical disease responsibilities. The Centers for Disease Control and Prevention also sponsors preventive services research.

[a] Abbreviations stand for Agency for Health Care Policy and Research, National Institute of Mental Health, National Institute on Drug Abuse, National Institute on Alcohol Abuse and Alcoholism, National Library of Medicine, Health Care Financing Administration/ Office of Research and Demonstrations, and Department of Veterans Affairs/Health Services Research and Development office, respectively.
[b] These figures represent AHCPR's total agency budget minus $2 million for "support."

SOURCE: Adapted from briefing materials distributed at the Association for Health Services Research Board of Directors meeting on February 14, 1995.

Federal support for health services research has been punctuated by periodic expressions of skepticism about its contributions (PSAC, 1972; Gray, 1992; see also Chapter 4). As this report was being drafted, the future of this support was once again in doubt (Brown, 1995). Even at current levels, funding for health services research is a smaller percentage of total health spending today than it was in 1970 (see Table 1.2).

TABLE 1.2 Federal Expenditures for Health Services Research in Relation to Total U.S. Health Spending, FY 1970 and FY 1994 (in millions of dollars)

Type of Expenditure	FY 1970	FY 1994[a]	% Change from 1970
Total U.S. health	$67,000	$1,000,000	1,393
Federal health	18,000	328,000	1,722
Federal biomedical research	1,600	10,000	525
Federal health services research	180	470	161
Federal health services research expenditures as percentage of U.S. total health expenditures	0.27	0.05	−81

[a]Not adjusted for inflation

SOURCE: Adapted from presentation by Clifton Gaus, Administrator of the Agency for Health Care Policy and Research, at the Association for Health Services Research Board of Directors meeting on February 14, 1995.

CONCLUSION

Health services research is a multidisciplinary field that investigates the structure, processes, and effects of health care services. It draws on a variety of clinical and academic disciplines and, at its most creative level, integrates their conceptual frameworks and methodologies to provide new ways of studying and understanding the health care system. The next chapter sets the context for the report's discussion of work force and training issues by reviewing the evolution of health services research as a field. It highlights areas of inquiry related to current controversies and developments, particularly those associated with managed care, integrated health systems, and other features of a health care system that is undergoing substantial restructuring.

2

Overview of Health Services Research

The field of health services research is just one outgrowth of scientific discoveries and technological innovations that have, in this century, transformed the understanding of the determinants of health and disease and allowed health workers to diagnose, prevent, and treat many conditions that once promised only death, disability, or discomfort. This transformation in the capabilities of medical care has provoked complex and continuing changes in the organization, cost, financing, governance, and social significance of health care in the United States.

Like higher income and education, greater access to health care has come to distinguish society's "haves" from its "have-nots." Health insurance has become the most valued employee benefit and a growing financial worry for many employers (IOM, 1993b). Efforts to assure universal access have created periodic upheavals in the political landscape, as have a succession of varied strategies to control spending on health care. These social, economic, and political developments have, in turn, helped to influence the direction and rate of changes in biomedical science and technology. Modern health services research was essentially born of demands for better understanding of how services are organized, financed, and delivered and with what consequences.

Recently, the health care system has been dramatically restructuring itself. Governments and employers have intensified their efforts to direct people into managed care plans that control patient access to practitioners and services, pay providers fixed amounts for a defined set of services to a defined set of patients, and otherwise manage the use and cost of care. Health care organizations are consolidating, expanding, shrinking, reorganizing, or otherwise changing in ways that are varied and often complex, and the power of specific institutions and professions is in flux. Health services research has played and will continue to play a central role in helping to document, assess, and explain these changes and their effects and to inform public and private decisions during a period of rapid change.

A BRIEF LOOK BACK

Although an extensive historical review was beyond the scope of this project, a brief look back is useful in understanding the field of health services research as it exists today. Not surprisingly, given the relatively imprecise boundaries of the field of health services research, any effort to trace its history involves some subjectivity, especially the further back in time one goes. Although the emphasis here is on the United States, it is clear that health services researchers from other countries have advanced the field in general and influenced American researchers. (The history of health service research education and training programs is considered in Chapter 4.)

The following historical overview notes several landmarks in the development of the field, including both advances in methodology and changes in the problems targeted for study.[1] It points out some of the contributions of health services research to policymaking or at least to policy debates. The review also highlights the critical role that federal funding for health services research has played in the development of the field.

Before 1965

Early instances of what may be broadly viewed as health services research tended to involve fairly simple descriptive surveys of personnel, facilities, or diseases. Starting with Michigan in 1883, states began to require the reporting of certain infectious conditions, and Congress in 1893 authorized the collection of such information from states and localities. Private organizations also became involved, as exemplified in the 1908 Chicago Medical Society birth record survey of midwifery, the first American Medical Association (AMA) survey of hospitals in 1909, and the 1914 AMA survey of state boards of health. Beginning in 1906 in Rochester, New York, dental inspections of school children

---

[1]This discussion draws on Somers and Somers, 1961; Anderson, 1968; PSAC, 1972; Flook and Sanazaro, 1973; NRC, 1977; IOM, 1979; Starr, 1982; Rorem, 1982; Shortell and Reinhardt, 1992; IOM, 1993b.

generated data that helped build understanding of the prevalence and variability of oral disease. These and similar kinds of data collection activities began to make clear the degree to which disease was associated with poverty. In the 1920s, the U.S. Public Health Service (PHS) continued investigations into the relationship between illness and income.

During the early years of this century, Ernest Codman pioneered empirical studies of the quality of medical care in hospitals. He argued that "hospitals, if they wish to be sure of improvement, must find out what their results are, must analyze their results, must compare their results with those of other hospitals" (Codman, 1914, cited in Fifer, 1990, p. 294). Codman analyzed 337 cases of hospital care, identifying errors of knowledge, judgment, and skill. Codman's analyses and arguments were highly influential on organizations such as the American College of Surgeons, although a concerted emphasis on evaluating care by its results or outcomes did not really take hold until relatively recently.

The work of the Committee on the Cost of Medical Care (CCMC) in the late 1920s and early 1930s became an early landmark in health services research, a truly multidisciplinary project in both its methods and its scope. With a research budget of $1 million, an astonishing figure for the time ($8.5 million in today's dollars), the 42-member committee and its 75-person staff produced 27 field studies and a final report between 1928 and 1932 (CCMC, 1932).[2] The CCMC studies and associated surveys provided the first extensive investigations of such matters as the incidence of illness and disability; the levels and kinds of care involved in treating specific illnesses and the implications for health work force and facilities planning; the distribution and organization of health care services; the level and types of health care expenditures; the uneven burden of medical expenses and access to medical care; and the development of group practice, prepayment, and other innovations in organizing and financing care. The scope and depth of the CCMC analyses have, arguably, not been approached again, and many subsequent analyses have come to generally similar conclusions, even several decades later.

In the 1930s, the federal Works Project Administration undertook the National Health Inventory, which was intended both to document health status in urban areas and to provide jobs for unemployed Americans. Except for limited state and supplementary studies, nothing as extensive was attempted until

---

[2] Six private foundations helped initiate the work of the CCMC: the Carnegie Corporation, the Josiah Macy, Jr., Foundation, the Milbank Memorial Fund, the Russell Sage Foundation, the Twentieth Century Fund, and the Julius Rosenwald Fund. Other organizations, including the AMA, also helped support the study with funding, information, or other assistance.

1956 when the National Health Survey Act (P.L. 84-652) authorized a continuing survey program supplemented by methodological and special topic studies.

In the private, nonprofit sector, the Health Insurance Plan of Greater New York and three Kaiser Permanente regions pioneered health services research in the group practice setting after the end of World War II (Densen, Shapiro, and Einhorn, 1959; Greenlick, Freenborn, and Pope, 1988). Beginning in the 1950s, some Blue Cross and Blue Shield plans also undertook applied health services research, for example to understand patterns of hospital use (Koen, 1965; Young, 1965).

One of the early federal government efforts to apply health services research in a systematic way to a problem in medical care organization came in the 1950s when funding was provided for internal PHS studies in hospital administration and for demonstration projects to improve hospital organization and design. These projects had been authorized by the 1948 Hospital Survey and Construction Act (P.L. 79-725), more commonly known as the Hill-Burton Act. In 1959, the Hospital Facilities Study Section of the PHS became the Health Services Research Study Section. In 1963, the Bureau of State Services in the Department of Health, Education and Welfare (DHEW) consolidated several research efforts and began the first organized extramural research program in community health services. During this period, some health services research was also being sponsored by the National Institutes of Health (NIH).

Indications that a coherent research field was emerging came with the creation of organizations, journals, and similar symbols. Within the American Public Health Association (APHA), the Medical Care Section (established by 1963) included a large contingent of health services researchers. The free-standing Association for Health Services Research (AHSR) was not, however, founded until 1981, when researchers recognized the value of having a focused voice for increased research funding (Gray, 1992) and a forum for bringing those with an interest in health services research together to share ideas and research.

Journals launched in the early 1960s included *Medical Care* (sponsored by the corresponding section of APHA), *Inquiry* (created by the Blue Cross and Blue Shield Association), and *Health Services Research* (established by Hospital Research and Education Trust, the research arm of the American Hospital Association). All are still being published today. In addition, more specialized journals often publish work that is based on health services research. These include the *Journal of Health Economics, Journal of Clinical Evaluation, Journal of Quality Improvement,* and *Journal of Outcomes Management,* as well as prominent clinical journals such as the *New England Journal of Medicine* and the *Journal of the American Medical Association.*

1965 and After

Federally Sponsored Research

In the 1960s, the federal government launched many significant initiatives in health care organization and financing, most notably Medicare and Medicaid. This expansion of government responsibility and spending focused policymakers' attention on the gaps in their knowledge about health care delivery and financing and about health behavior. It highlighted the need for efforts to evaluate the impacts of government programs and the factors contributing to the strengths, weaknesses, and unanticipated consequences of these programs. In addition, 1966 legislation authorizing the comprehensive Neighborhood Health Center component of the Office of Economic Opportunity (OEO) launched a large number of community health centers and a subsequent OEO effort to evaluate their community impact.

National Center for Health Services Research. In 1965, the White House Conference on Health recommended the creation of a National Institute of Community Health Services to coordinate and stimulate health services research related to these and other federal health interests. Subsequently, the 1967 *Report to the President on Medical Care Prices* recommended a role for a national center in conducting research on cost containment, prepaid group practice, and community health care systems (Flook and Sanazaro, 1973).

In 1967, Congress enacted P.L. 90-174, which authorized the PHS to undertake a range of research, demonstration, and training activities. Under this general authority, the Secretary of DHEW established the National Center for Health Services Research and Development (NCHSR).[3] NCHSR consolidated research activities from several units of DHEW, including those units concerned with community health service, medical care administration, and hospital and medical facilities. In addition, NCHSR established several health services research centers through contracts with academic or other outside organizations, including Harvard University, the University of California, Los Angeles; the University of North Carolina; and Kaiser Permanente in Northern and Southern California. Successor agencies have continued to use the "centers" concept in various forms with various participants.

---

[3]In conjunction with various governmental reorganizations, the National Center was variously renamed the Bureau of Health Services Research, the Bureau of Health Services Research and Evaluation, and the National Center for Health Services Research (IOM, 1979). The National Center was absorbed into the Agency for Health Care Policy and Research in 1989.

After 1969, NCHSR increasingly focused its resources on relatively short-term research and development (R&D) projects rather than on longer-term research. The goal was to identify, design, develop, introduce, test, evaluate, and replicate new health services strategies that met "specified performance criteria under realistic operating conditions" (Flook and Sanazaro, 1973, p. 158). The initial target areas for R&D activities were

- physician and dentist extenders,
- cost containment and financing,
- quality of care,
- medical technology, and
- health data systems.

Experience acquired in two of these R&D areas had particular policy significance in the 1970s. In the quality arena, the Experimental Medical Care Review Organization program developed and partially tested the structures and processes for quality assurance that became the basis for the Professional Standards Review Organization program, created in 1972 mainly for the Medicare program. In the data systems area, the Health Services Foundation of the Blue Cross Association carried out demonstration projects in the 1970s to test a uniform hospital discharge data set. This work influenced the creation of a cooperative federal-state-local health statistics system overseen by the National Center for Health Statistics, which itself had been created in 1974 (NRC and IOM, 1992).

In 1989, NCHSR was absorbed into the Agency for Health Care Policy and Research (AHCPR). The legislation that established the AHCPR focused the agency's activities on effectiveness research, technology assessment, and guidelines for clinical practice.[4] The selection of these areas reflected policymakers' frustrations with continually escalating health care costs and their general awareness of two decades of health services research that had (1) documented wide variations in medical practices (e.g., Wennberg and Gittelsohn, 1982; Wennberg, 1984; Brook, Chassin, Park, et al., 1986), (2) suggested that some health care services were of little or no value (e.g, Chassin, Kosecoff, Park, et al., 1987; Eddy and Billings, 1988), and (3) examined various kinds of economic and organizational incentives to reduce inappropriate variation and utilization (e.g., Ellwood, 1975, 1988; Eisenberg, 1986; Enthoven, 1988).

Health Care Financing Administration. The Health Care Financing Administration (HCFA), which was established in 1974, also developed an extensive array of research activities, in particular through its Office of Research

---

[4]See Gray (1992) for an interesting account of the agency's creation.

and Demonstrations. This office built on the work of the Office of Research and Statistics in the Social Security Administration, which initially administered the Medicare program.

In the late 1970s, HCFA was the major funder of research on health insurance and health care expenditures (IOM, 1979). The agency also initiated demonstration projects to examine enrollment, payment, benefit design, and other issues involved in extending health maintenance organization (HMO) coverage to Medicare beneficiaries and to test a model of capitated acute and long-term care for frail older persons with a special emphasis on geriatrics (Langwell, Rossiter, Brown, et al., 1987; Harrington and Newcomer, 1991; Kane and Blewett, 1993).

In addition, HCFA (sometimes building on work initially funded by NCHSR) has supported research to develop methods to pay for services to Medicare and Medicaid beneficiaries in ways that would encourage cost-effective health care by discouraging unnecessary use of inpatient care, expensive technologies, and specialist services. The initials for the resulting tools—in particular, DRGs (for prospective payment for hospitals based on diagnosis-related groups), RBRVS (for physician payment based on a resource-based relative value scale), and AAPCC (for a risk-adjusted, capitated payment for health care plans)—have become part of the everyday vocabulary of policymakers and managers. The development of better methods for adjusting payments for services to account for a patient's health status—or risk of incurring expenses—is a major issue on HCFA's current research agenda.

Department of Veterans Affairs. As directed by Congress, the Department of Veterans Affairs (VA) has had a health services research and development office, referred to as HSR&D, since 1976. In 1981, the office was "reoriented to emphasize health services research as a management tool" to improve health care for veterans (Goldschmidt, 1986, p. 798). As part of this initiative, the VA set up research field offices in each of its six regions. It also established several Centers for Cooperative Studies in Health Services, which provide support to investigators planning large-scale studies and promote collaborative use of common research protocols and data sets. In addition, the VA has funded the Management Decision Research Center, which provides consultation, technical assistance, and research support to improve system level management and the capabilities of VA senior staff. Recently, in conjunction with the Foundation for Health Services Research, the VA launched a new periodic publication, *Forum: Translating Research into Quality Health Care for Veterans.*

Other federal agencies. In addition to the units cited above, several other federal agencies developed health services research agendas. For example, the Office of Economic Opportunity initiated (but only briefly oversaw) the national

Health Insurance Study at the RAND Corporation in 1971. This project became the Health Insurance Experiment (HIE), which "remains one of the largest and longest-running social science research projects ever completed" (Newhouse and the Insurance Experiment Group, 1993, p. vii). It continued into the late 1980s with support from the Office of the Assistant Secretary for Planning and Evaluation in the Department of Health and Human Services. Several institutes of the NIH have also supported health services research. Most notable are the institutes concerned with mental health, drug abuse, and alcoholism and alcohol abuse, which are currently mandated to set aside 15 percent of their budgets for health services research. Other parts of the NIH and the Departments of Agriculture, Defense, Education, and Energy also have sponsored some activities that could be counted as health services research, although they may not be explicitly described as such.[5]

Other Sponsors of Health Services Research

Private foundations, state governments, industry, and other sources have also supported health services research, although specific data on the level and distribution of such funding are largely unavailable. The HSRProj database maintained by the National Library of Medicine, however, provides some information on foundation funding of health services research studies. An analysis of roughly 900 of the 1,200 studies[6] listed in the database late in 1994, showed that six private foundations (the Robert Wood Johnson Foundation, W.K. Kellogg Foundation, Pew Charitable Trusts, John A. Hartford Foundation, Commonwealth Fund, and Henry J. Kaiser Family Foundation) provided approximately 20 percent ($70 million) of the funding for the studies listed; the federal government provided the other 80 percent. HSRProj does not contain information on the research supported by state governments or industry.

Several private foundations, including those that funded the work of the CCMC between 1928 and 1932, have a long history of funding health services research. Examples of major foundation-sponsored research activities include projects on the appropriateness of medical care (e.g., work at RAND sponsored by the Commonwealth Fund and others), indicators of health status (e.g., IOM conferences on advances in health status assessment funded by the Henry J.

---

[5]For example, the National Institute of Nursing Research technically does not fund health services research. Some of the nursing research projects they support do, however, seek to increase knowledge of the structure, processes, and effects of health services—specifically, nursing services—for individuals and populations.

[6]Data elements were missing on 300 of the files. The committee could not determine if the missing files contained information on foundation- or government-funded studies.

Kaiser Family Foundation), and regional data projects (e.g., work supported by the John A. Hartford Foundation).

The committee is aware of few states that undertake or sponsor significant health services research on an ongoing basis, and much of the research on state programs and problems is actually sponsored by the federal government or private foundations. States, however, have undertaken analytic work to support policy decisions on a variety of health problems or issues including infant mortality, use of managed care arrangements for Medicaid beneficiaries, nursing home regulation, substance abuse, and access for underserved populations. They often contract on an ad hoc basis with consulting firms, research organizations, or universities for studies of specific programs or issues. Some notable examples of state-supported health services research include the New York State Department of Health's analyses of physician-specific mortality rates for cardiac surgery (Hannan, Kilburn, Racz, et al., 1994; Green and Whitfield, 1995) and the work of the Oregon Health Resources Commission to develop a priority list or rank ordering of combinations of medical conditions and treatments as a basis for allocating limited resources for health care (Eddy, 1991).

In the past 50 years, various private organizations have created (and sometimes abolished) research arms to conduct both externally and internally sponsored research. These include professional associations (e.g., the American Hospital Association, the AMA), insurers (e.g, individual Blue Cross and Blue Shield plans), community health groups (e.g., Greater Detroit Area Health Council), and prepaid group health plans (e.g., the Health Insurance Plan of Greater New York, Group Health Cooperative of Puget Sound, Kaiser Permanente). The research funding pattern found in early prepaid group practice plans appears typical of this larger group of organizations. That is, the organizations provided seed money, but the majority of the funding for research came from the federal government. Over a 30-year period, for example, Kaiser Permanente contributed approximately $25 million, or 16 percent, of the $150 million in total funding for its Northwest region's Center for Health Services Research.

How much private organizations, including competing health plans, will invest in health services research in the future is an important question. When they invest, business considerations will guide their choices of topics and their decisions about making information publicly available. For example, health plans that support technology assessments to inform coverage or influence practice patterns may conclude that subjecting their scientific analyses to peer review and public scrutiny provides essential credibility. Similarly, in some situations, the competitive advantage is in having early access to information for decisionmaking, and once this time-limited benefit has been reaped, the information may be made public. In other cases, commercial considerations may be weighed differently. For example, some systems to assess severity of illness have kept some of their algorithms proprietary while making other elements public (IOM, 1989). Firms that provide services such as technology assessments on a subscription basis typically have to limit public availability of their analyses or find other ways of generating income for the activity. Market research on consumer attitudes and decisionmaking is traditionally proprietary, although purchasers are now demanding that some information about consumer satisfaction with competitive health plans be made public.

Public and private universities have received much of the extramural health services research funds provided by federal agencies, and they also have obtained research funding from private foundations and industry. In addition, universities have sometimes provided seed grants or have self-funded a small amount of health services research from their own resources. The committee was not aware of any systematic information on the extent of university-sponsored (as opposed to university-conducted) research.

Several freestanding private research organizations, such as the Urban Institute, Lewin-VHI, Abt Associates, Mathematica Policy Research, and Battelle Memorial Institute, have been major recipients of public and private research funds and have made significant contributions to health services research. The RAND Corporation, as already mentioned, conducted the multi-million-dollar national HIE as well as several of the studies of appropriate medical care cited earlier. As far as the committee is aware, however, these organizations are able to undertake little if any self-funded research.

HEALTH SERVICES RESEARCH TODAY AND TOMORROW

As a multidisciplinary field, health services research has drawn on and combined concepts and methods from many disciplines to provide frameworks for analyzing the structures, processes, and outcomes of health care and for informing decisionmaking. The agenda of topics for future research is quite lengthy and challenging. It both builds on longstanding questions about the availability, effectiveness, and cost of health care and incorporates new emphases that reflect the complex changes now occurring in the health care system. The extent to which this research agenda can be implemented depends significantly on the level and stability of federal funding, which has been and continues to be uncertain.

The discussion of health research issues below is quite selective, but it illustrates the central themes of the field: the organization and financing of health services; access to health care; practitioner, patient, and consumer behavior; quality of care; clinical evaluation and outcomes research; informatics and clinical decisionmaking; and the health professions work force. Although categorizations of research areas inevitably emphasize separation, cross-cutting inquiry is an important characteristic of the field.

Organization and Financing of Health Services

The recent debate over health care reform has highlighted concerns about the organization and financing of health care that health services researchers have long studied. Although it may have been largely invisible to the public, the media, and many political figures, three decades of health service research clearly contributed to the formulation of recent proposals for health care reform. This contribution is reflected in the prominence in reform proposals of provisions involving managed care, consumer choice, outcomes and performance monitoring, and risk selection in health insurance—even though researchers might sometimes disagree with the policy conclusions set forth in specific proposals.

Health services research has helped to clarify the features and effects of health insurance and market-based strategies of health care (e.g., requiring patients to bear some of the economic cost of their health care decisions and offering choices among health plans). In particular, it has shed more light on a dilemma long familiar to actuaries: that consumers' continuing exercise of choice in the purchase of health insurance can seriously diminish the degree to which the burden of health care expenses is shared among the well and the ill and thus undermine the very notion of insurance. Various studies (many sponsored by HCFA as part of its effort to direct Medicare beneficiaries into HMOs) have underscored how the financial benefits to health plans of avoiding high-risk individuals could be far greater than the rewards from cost-effective management of health care and have highlighted how difficult it is to compensate for this risk selection dynamic (IOM, 1993). Although other considerations and values certainly shaped the debate over health care reform, concern about insurance dynamics was central to controversies about minimum or standardized benefit packages, health insurance purchasing cooperatives, community- versus experience-based pricing of insurance, statewide reinsurance pools, medical savings plans, and regulation of marketing practices.

Health services research has illuminated the incentives of traditional fee-for-service and cost-based mechanisms for paying for health care. It has also devised tools and techniques that have facilitated the development of various alternative methods of paying for health services. As described earlier, these mechanisms include case-based payment for hospital services related to broad diagnostic groups, relative value scales for individual physician services, and adjusted per capita payments to health care organizations responsible for enrolled populations.

As more health services have shifted from the hospital to other settings, researchers have attempted to evaluate the effects of these shifts on the quality, cost, and availability of care. Similarly, researchers continue to investigate the extent to which care provided by dental hygienists, nurse practitioners, occupational therapists, physical therapists, physician assistants, and other "mid-level" practitioners can safely, effectively, and efficiently substitute for physician and dentist care. These discussions have focused attention on conceptual and methodological questions about what constitutes effective care and who experiences the costs or savings of alternative modes of care.

Access to Health Care

In the health care context, access may be defined as the timely receipt of appropriate care (IOM, 1993a). From the field's earliest days, access has been an important focus of health services research, which has drawn attention to differences in access across income, racial, and other groups. Although it has helped to identify the cultural, organizational, and other nonfinancial barriers to access, it has particularly highlighted the financial barriers including the lack of insurance coverage.

Research has delineated who is less likely to have health insurance and how coverage affects access to care, utilization of services, and health outcomes. It has clarified the central role played by employers, especially larger employers, in insuring full-time, full-year workers and their families. Each year, new survey results are closely examined for changes in the numbers and proportion of uninsured in the population. Researchers continue to explore how lack of coverage affects health, for example, by investigating the impact of cutbacks in Medicaid coverage (Lurie, Ward, Shapiro, et al., 1984; Hadley, Steinberg, and Feder, 1991). Such research can inform both the public and policymakers and shape governmental or political decisions.

Quality of Care

With rising costs have come demands for greater accountability from health care practitioners and institutions and for monitoring tools or systems that will document the quality of care. Quality has been defined in another IOM study as "the degree to which health services for individuals and populations increase the likelihood of desired health outcomes and are consistent with current professional knowledge" (1990b, p. 21). Health services researchers attempt to define and identify quality problems such as unnecessary or inappropriate care, underuse of appropriate care, and poor technical or interpersonal care. Drawing on concepts and techniques from industrial quality management, statistics, informatics, and operations research, health services researchers have been investigating strategies for monitoring performance and strengthening accountability. They have developed methods to measure health outcomes and to link variations in outcomes to characteristics of health care. Researchers have also sought to educate potential users—consumers, purchasers, and policymakers—about the strengths and limitations of specific monitoring and accountability mechanisms.

One critical need is for continued development and testing of practical and economical mechanisms for collecting, synthesizing, and disseminating valid, reliable, and usable health data. For example, researchers have investigated how "report cards" might be designed and implemented to help purchasers and consumers choose among health plans or providers. Laying a data-driven foundation for such judgments involves applied, theoretical, and philosophical challenges for research and policy in both public and private spheres.

A particular challenge involves methods for assuring that performance comparisons reflect appropriate adjustments for different patient populations. Despite considerable progress, developing techniques to adjust for differences in severity of illness, comorbidity, and other factors continues to be among most difficult technical problems facing health services research today. These problems are, in many respects, another manifestation of those facing health plans when they enroll sicker populations that make their costs higher than those of competitors with healthier enrollees.

Health services researchers can also inform (but not decide) the debate over the merits of governmental versus market strategies for monitoring and improving quality. Research in the 1970s contributed to skepticism about the effectiveness of community health planning, professional review organizations, and other regulatory strategies for improving efficiency and quality in health care. Now that market-driven strategies predominate, the focus of research is shifting. One concern is whether adequate tools and the data are at hand to assess the effects of a restructured health care system, especially when the incentives for providing too much care are diminishing and those for providing too little care are increasing.

Although some role for external monitoring is generally conceded, many believe that quality improvement must, for the most part, be internally motivated and managed (IOM, 1990b). That means that large health care organizations need not only leadership but also people and continuing processes for establishing objectives, designing strategies for meeting those objectives, implementing the strategies, collecting and analyzing evidence about their impact, and redesigning activities as appropriate. In this environment, the boundaries of research, management, and marketing can become blurred.

Clinical Evaluation and Outcomes Research

New medical technologies are often put into practice without valid evaluations of their effectiveness or their cost-effectiveness (OTA, 1994). Moreover, some long-standing practices depend on unverified claims of efficacy (expected benefit under ideal conditions of use) and effectiveness (expected benefit under average conditions of use). Dissatisfaction with these circumstances has given rise to clinical evaluative studies and outcomes research on the benefits and harms of different strategies for preventing, diagnosing, or treating illness. Relevant studies have focused on the assessment and comparison of alternative interventions for a given clinical problem and the identification of short-term and long-term outcomes of interest to patients, practitioners, and policymakers. In addition, researchers have devised instruments or techniques for measuring a variety of health outcomes, comparing the performance of health care organizations, and accounting for patient characteristics and other variables that may complicate comparisons of outcomes.

The scope of clinical evaluations and outcomes studies is wide. Examples include evaluations of oral health outcomes in countries with different approaches to preventing and treating oral disease and organizing oral health services, assessments of the effectiveness of home-based intervention for people caring for a family member with dementia, and studies of whether treatment for skin ulcers in people with diabetes varies according to the type of doctor seen. More generally, the health outcomes of interest to practitioners, patients, and other decisions are quite diverse. They include not only mortality and morbidity but also health status, functional capacities, quality of life, patient and family satisfaction with health services, and professional satisfaction.

The measurement of health status and functional outcomes comprises a major area needing further theoretical development, which could include development of a "production function" for health. That would require economists, clinicians, and others to collaborate on the design of integrated health systems that will economically produce the health outcomes that are desired by patients and their families. There are few data or theories to clarify the trade-offs between costs and quality.

The results of clinical evaluations and outcomes research may be used in formulating clinical practice guidelines to assist patients and providers in making decisions about appropriate medical care (IOM, 1992). More generally, translating evaluative and outcomes knowledge into improved medical care and its outcomes will require contributions from other areas of health services research including those concerned with practitioner and patient decisionmaking, medical informatics, and quality improvement strategies.

Informatics and Clinical Decisionmaking

The country has made large investments in medical information systems that are supplying health care providers, managers, and researchers with quicker and easier access to more complete health care information about both individuals and groups. The information provided by computer-based information systems is proving particularly useful for clinicians, administrators, and researchers who are attempting to measure and improve the quality and cost-effectiveness of health services through better design and management of clinical and administrative systems. Important challenges for health services researchers, computer scientists, and others remain in such areas as linking patient records across inpatient and outpatient care settings; establishing protocols for ensuring the confidentiality and accuracy of information; and developing more user-friendly hardware and software for entering, retrieving, or analyzing information. In these activities, the federally sponsored National Information Infrastructure initiative will permit a wide variety of parties, including health services researchers, to transmit, store, process, analyze, and display data in different forms such as text, still images, sound, and video (Lasker, Humphreys, and Braithewaite, 1995).

Clinicians have access to a variety of on-line and other information resources. They may, for example, subscribe to on-line article retrieval services such as Medline and Grateful Med, as well as the other specialized medical information services provided by the National Library of Medicine. They may also purchase CD-ROM or other software packages that allow them to search the medical literature for information on specific clinical problems, to locate clinical practice guidelines, and to work through quantitative algorithms to identify probabilities of various benefits or harms of alternative clinical strategies for a given patient's problem. Patients also have access to much of this information and may use it to guide their own decisions—with or without consulting a clinician. The impact of these information resources on attitudes and behavior will present new research questions in an area of long-standing interest to health services researchers.

In addition to providing information, computer-based information systems can incorporate a variety of tools to assist clinical decisionmaking. These tools include automatic reminders or alerts that are triggered when certain patient information is entered or obtained or when certain pharmacy, laboratory, or other tests are ordered. Thus, a physician or nurse may be reminded that a diabetic patient is due for an opthalmalogic test or that penicillin is contraindicated for a patient with a past allergic reaction to the drug. The development and evaluation of these decision aids pose important opportunities for health services researchers.

Practitioner, Patient, and Consumer Behavior

Health services and behavioral science researchers have spent many years exploring health-related human behavior and studying how practitioners and patients make decisions about health and health care. Investigators continue to search for the demographic, cultural, economic, and other factors that shape individual actions such as seeking medical or dental care, selecting among treatment options, following treatment recommendations, and purchasing health insurance (or selecting from alternative insurance plans). Much, however, remains to be learned about ways of encouraging desired patient behaviors and decisions on such diverse subjects as adherence to dietary protocols for diabetes, timely and continuing use of preventive services, and appropriate requests for antibiotics.

Research on practitioner behavior likewise continues. Investigators ask how education, training, professional socialization, practice environments, economic incentives, and other factors affect decisions. They raise challenging issues such as how to reconcile dramatic variations in rates of health care interventions with the notion that there is a common base of professional knowledge accessible to all practitioners. Do management models that stress the reduction of such variations promise—particularly in a competitive market—to support or undermine the role of the clinician as an expert agent and advocate for patient interests? In a restructured health care system, managers can look to past research on physician responses to economic incentives, guidelines for clinical practice, data on practice patterns, and other management or policy tools.

Health Professions Work Force

Some of the most sensitive questions asked of health services researchers involve the education and supply of health care workers. Are there too many nurses or are there too few? Does the country have too few generalist practitioners or too many specialists or both? Are health professionals located appropriately across geographic areas? How will the changing medical marketplace affect demand for health personnel and for health professions education programs? Should the content of medical education change? What attracts qualified people to particular professions? What are the obstacles to increased participation by underrepresented minorities in the health care work force?

Efforts by analysts and policymakers to forecast and plan the supply of health personnel and services have not proved particularly successful (Feil, Welch, and Fisher, 1993; Kindig, 1994; Capilouto, Capilouto, and Ohsfeldt,

1995; IOM, 1995). Health services researchers are, however, continuing efforts to improve their estimating tools (NRC, 1994). These difficulties and efforts, which obviously are significant for this study, are discussed further in Chapter 3.

CONCLUSION

The discussion above has several implications for the education and training issues that this IOM committee was asked to examine. First, health service researchers face no shortage of important, contentious questions and methodologic challenges. Second, despite some skepticism, public and private decisionmakers have for decades been influenced by health services research (although they may not have known the source for what has become common knowledge), and they have increasingly looked to it for tools to help measure the effectiveness of health services and organizations. This implies some trajectory of rising demand for research and people to design, conduct, and report it. Third, demands for internal management information and external accountability should provide employment opportunities for health services researchers as large medical care organizations, integrated health systems, and accrediting agencies establish health services research units to provide information and analyses. Fourth, public resources for health services research are vulnerable when attempts are made to pare government budgets, which complicates efforts to determine how many health services researchers should be trained. Fifth, research questions that have a public good aspect may be less likely be addressed by market organizations if they cannot readily capture the major benefit of their research investment.

The next chapter of this report discusses the health services research work force in more detail. It also presents what the committee learned about public and private demand for health services research and researchers.

3

The Health Services Research Work Force

To a greater degree than is true of many professions requiring postbaccalaureate education, health services researchers are defined by their work, not by their degrees. Physicians, nurses, and dentists, in contrast, are identified by their degrees, even when they are not actively practicing. Furthermore, although some health services researchers have degrees in the field of health services research, many have disciplinary degrees in public health, sociology, economics, or other fields. They may identify themselves as much with their discipline as with the field of health services research, perhaps because the field is relatively young.

The health services research work force is marked by diversity along many dimensions. It includes individuals with widely varying backgrounds—social scientists, behavioral scientists, statisticians, public health specialists, physicians, nurses—who come to the field by many different educational paths. These paths include master's, doctoral, and clinical degrees as well as fellowships, on-the-job training, and summer or other short-term programs.

Employment settings are also varied and include universities, academic health centers, government agencies, health care delivery and insurance organizations, consulting firms, and freestanding research organizations. Some organizations employ more than 100 health services researchers; others choose to contract for all or most of the research they need. Many organizations employ a wide variety of types and levels of researchers, who frequently work as teams. Such teams may include clinicians and master's-level and doctoral-level researchers who have backgrounds in such diverse areas as internal medicine, nursing, health economics, epidemiology, and health care administration. In addition to working as members of multidisciplinary teams, individual researchers must, in many cases, consider the perspectives of multiple disciplines in their own particular research projects.

As described in Chapter 1, the health services research work force has three components: (1) investigators who originate, design, supervise, and report basic and applied health services research; (2) researchers who assist in the conduct of health services research under the direction of others; and (3) individuals who analyze information and apply the tools of health services research in management and policy settings. The first group is composed largely of individuals with research doctorates; the latter two groups include many with master's-level education. Depending on their level of education, experience, and interest in health services research, clinicians may be found in all three groups.

This chapter presents the results of this committee's efforts to identify and describe the work force, to relate current supply to demand, and to project future trends. The discussion illustrates the complexities created by the multidisciplinary character of the field, its relative youth, and the diversity of its membership.

THE CURRENT WORK FORCE

A major objective of the current study was a more comprehensive count of current health services researchers than has been available in the past. The database compiled for this report will provide others with a starting point for more detailed surveys of work force characteristics, career paths, and other important information.

Methodological Issues

Any effort to count and describe the health services research work force must overcome several challenges. First, because the field is multidisciplinary rather than marked by a defining degree, discipline, or credential, it is not readily tracked in yearly censuses or biennial sample surveys of individuals who have earned or are working toward doctoral degrees.[1] These data are a major

---

[1]The National Research Council (NRC) administers the Survey of Doctorate Recipients, a longitudinal sample survey that began in 1973. The data are collected by the NRC on behalf of the National Science Foundation. Samples are based on a yearly doctorate census that the NRC has administered since 1958. In alternate years, samples are drawn either humanities' doctorates or science and engineering doctorates. Those selected are then reinterviewed until they reach age 70, die, or drop out of the survey. Although certain categories of individuals who *might* be health services researchers (e.g.,

resource for those attempting to determine the supply of researchers in a field and describe their demographic characteristics, employment status, and career paths. Other databases such as those maintained by the American Medical Association also lack codes that would identify health services researchers.

A second and related difficulty is that academic researchers, a major component of most research work forces, are not concentrated in identifiable health services research programs. Rather, they are widely scattered across a variety of disciplinary departments (e.g., economics, sociology), professional schools (e.g., medicine, dentistry, business, nursing), and variably named health-related programs (e.g., health policy, health administration). Even in more traditional fields, it is "surprisingly difficult" to compile reliable information on faculty positions and openings (Browne, 1995, p. 16).

Third, the major professional organization for the field, the Association for Health Services Research (AHSR), is relatively young and small. Compared to larger and longer-established professions and disciplines, it has limited personnel and employment databases. The American Mathematical Society and the American Institute of Physics, in contrast, survey new doctoral recipients each summer and then resurvey them in the spring to determine their employment status, and the American Chemical Society recently undertook a survey to help assess unemployment and underemployment (Browne, 1995; COSEPUP, 1995).

Committee Data Collection Strategies

To identify members of the health services research work force, the committee used two different strategies: one that combined existing data sources and the other that collected new information. (See Appendix A for more details on the work, which was supported by the Robert Wood Johnson Foundation and the Baxter Foundation and was carried out in early 1995 by the Wisconsin Network for Health Policy Research at the University of Wisconsin–Madison.) The *first strategy* was to combine lists of health services researchers from a variety of sources, most notably, the membership list of the AHSR[2] and the list

---

those awarded doctorates in public health, biostatistics, or epidemiology) are categorized, the survey is of little use for identifying new entrants to the field of health service research. NRC staff report that health services research has not met their criterion for adding a category to the survey. That criterion requires that at least ten survey recipients in each of the past three surveys identify the category in the space provided for "other" fields to be mentioned.

[2]This listing excludes individuals who take advantage of an employer's institutional membership, which provides AHSR benefits—such as discounted registration for the annual meeting—to up to 10 individuals from the member institution.

of principal investigators in HSRProj, the National Library of Medicine database of funded health services research projects. To these lists were added names from brochures of about 50 health research centers and names from other, smaller lists, including those participating in recent AHSR annual meetings and members of the Sigma Theta Tau, the nursing research honorary society. This combined database is the most comprehensive listing of health services researchers to date. It contains the following information (if available) for each individual: degree, address, name of employer, and telephone number.

The *second strategy* involved new data collection through a survey of organizational employers of health services researchers (see Appendix A for more details). This survey was sent to nearly 500 organizations identified from AHSR records and other sources. It asked respondents to provide information about their health services researchers, their current and future research priorities, and current and future hiring. The categories of organizations that received the survey included university-based research centers, private research organizations and think tanks, research units in health plans, managed care organizations, insurance companies, pharmaceutical companies, and federal and state government agencies. Although the Wisconsin group and this committee believe that these organizations represent a large percentage of major employers of health services researchers, no data are available to document the survey's comprehensiveness or representativeness. Moreover, the response rate for the survey was only 31 percent so the committee interpreted the results with caution.

To strengthen its qualitative understanding of the demand for health services researchers, the committee also conducted telephone interviews with 28 individuals representing several categories of health-related organizations including insurers, pharmaceutical companies, integrated health systems, state government agencies, and consulting firms. (Although the committee made an effort to contact a range of organizations, those participating were not a random sample, and responses may not be representative of the larger universe of organizations.) Questions focused on the type of issues currently being studied or considered for study in the next five years, the number and type of researchers employed, and experience in recruiting well-qualified candidates.

Size and Characteristics of the Work Force

The database that resulted from the two data collection strategies described above includes information on 4,920 health services researchers. Information on the type of degrees earned was available for just under two-thirds of those listed. Of these, 49 percent were reported as having Ph.D.s (or, in a relatively small number of cases, Sc.D.s or Ed.D.s). Clinicians accounted for about 28 percent of the group, and more than three-quarters of these were physicians.

Geographically, 27 percent of the researchers in the database are located in the South Atlantic region of the country, primarily because of the concentration of researchers in Maryland and the District of Columbia. The next highest concentrations of health services researchers are seen in the Pacific region (16 percent) and the East North Central region (16 percent). California, with 567 health services researchers, has the largest state contingent, followed by Maryland (423), the District of Columbia (321), Massachusetts (317), and Pennsylvania (305).

As far as the committee could ascertain, only one survey of health services researchers, which was conducted in 1978 by a special National Research Council (NRC) panel, has attempted to describe the work force in more detail. That study (Ebert–Flattau and Perkoff, 1983) identified two populations of researchers. The first group, principal investigators, was older and more than 90 percent were male; more than one-third held medical degrees and two-fifths had research doctorates. The second group, former trainees (i.e., recipients of health services research traineeships), was younger and nearly one-half were female; two-thirds held research doctorates but only one-tenth held a medical degree (NRC, 1981, p. 107). Both groups were overwhelmingly Caucasian, but the trainee group was somewhat less so (94 percent versus 97 percent). More than three-quarters of each category were engaged at some level in health services research. The percentage of time spent in research (as opposed to management or other activities) was lower than for biomedical researchers but higher than for behavioral science researchers. About 66 percent were employed in academic institutions, and about 4 percent of former trainees and 11 percent of investigators were employed in business or industry (not including health care delivery). Unemployment was very low (2 percent).

Based on its familiarity with the health services research community (but lacking explicit information from the researcher database), the committee believes it likely that women are better represented in the class of principal investigators than in the 1978 survey, although they probably remain a minority. As in 1978, clinicians (especially physicians) appear to remain more common in the leadership segment of the research work force than in health services research as a whole. (For example, in 1995, more than one-third of the members of the Boards of the AHSR and the Foundation for Health Services Research (FHSR), had clinical degrees. At the association's 1995 annual meeting, 6 of the 11 individuals featured in "meet-the-expert" sessions were clinicians.)

No reliable longitudinal data on the health services research work force are available. Certainly, AHSR membership, both individual and organizational, has grown—from 450 individual and 25 organizational members in 1983 to 2,248 individual members and 128 organizational members in 1994. Such membership figures, however, constitute an unsatisfactory measure of overall work force size and growth for a number of reasons. Not all AHSR members are producers of health services research; some are users of this research (e.g., public and private sector administrators, students, journal editors and writers).[3] In addition, some health services researchers may not hold individual membership in AHSR if they are affiliated with organizations that hold institutional memberships, and some individuals will choose not to join, perhaps because they already belong to several other professional groups. Once created, an organization can expect fast growth as it draws from an existing pool of potential members. Even later, when a greater proportion of new members will be new entrants to the field, some new members will be established researchers who have, for one reason or another, finally decided to join the organization. In sum, AHSR membership is not a good indicator of the size of the health services research work force or its growth.

Supply in Relation to Demand

The data gathered by the committee did not allow quantitative assessments of the relationship between the current supply of and demand for health services researchers. For example, the committee found no recent statistics on unemployment and underemployment rates, salary trends, or job vacancy rates for health services researchers. Qualitative information suggested healthy demand for researchers in academic settings (e.g., clinical departments that have added health services research to their research portfolio) and private sector organizations (e.g, health plans or insurers that have recently created or strengthened research units).

The committee also found some qualitative evidence of demand pressure in certain areas. Overall, more than half of the 154 responding organizations in the employer mail survey indicated that they have had difficulty recruiting certain types of health services researchers in the last few years. The areas most frequently mentioned were outcomes and health status measurement, health economics, biostatistics, epidemiology, and health policy analysis. (See Appendix A for a discussion of this survey and its limitations.)

These results of the written survey (which as previously noted had a low response rate) were reinforced by telephone interviews conducted by the committee with representatives of health-related organizations. In these interviews, committee members heard of problems in recruiting well-trained and experienced researchers in health economics, epidemiology, database management, biostatistics, psychometrics, and organizational behavior. Those

---

[3]In recent years, the AHSR has attempted to identify such individuals by asking member applicants to indicate whether or not they consider themselves health services researchers. As described in Appendix A, the database created for this study excludes those who answered "no" to this question.

with experience in state government noted that the demand from state administrative and legislative offices was not for academically oriented researchers but for people prepared to conduct policy analyses and interpret research findings in the "real world" of policymaking. Executives in health care financing organizations mentioned that researchers with work experience in managed care or research management were hard to find. Several employers mentioned that they receive weekly calls from "headhunters" looking to recruit researchers with the backgrounds mentioned above. Some indicated that they look for people who have experience in health services and that they are generally indifferent to candidates' specific degrees. Others indicated that they looked for people who are well-trained in specific disciplines because they feel that knowledge about health services can be taught on the job.

THE FUTURE WORK FORCE

Estimating the Future Supply of Personnel

To develop a rough estimate of the health services research pipeline, the committee combined information found in the 1991–1992 FHSR directory of graduate programs with responses to its own canvass of these programs. (See Appendix B for more details.) For the 76 respondents whose responses updated the FHSR directory information, the committee used their report of the number of students enrolled in each class. For the 45 respondents who did not return the update, the committee used the enrollment information reported in the 1991–1992 FHSR directory. (For those who responded, the committee compared the updated and earlier figures and found little change in enrollments for most programs, but the pattern for nonrespondents might be different.)

The combined figures on enrollment in each class from the two data sources show approximately 1,015 master's students, 511 students in doctoral programs, and 197 individuals in postdoctoral fellowships. As an estimate of the health services research pipeline, this number must be interpreted cautiously. On the one hand, for the master's level and other programs that offer concentrations in areas in addition to health services research, the numbers may include students who have concentrations other than health services research. On the other hand, the numbers refer to enrollments in *each class* not to *total* enrollments.[4]

---

[4]By way of contrast, for medical and dental schools, enrollments are reported separately for the first through fourth years of school as well as for those graduating in a year. To obtain an estimate of total enrollment, the committee considered multiplying the enrollment figure for each program by the reported years to complete a degree—two years for most master's-level programs and four to five years for doctoral programs. If

Beyond attempting to identify researchers in training, projecting the future supply of researchers is a considerably more difficult task than counting current researchers in any field or discipline. For its 1994 report, the NRC Committee on National Needs for Biomedical and Behavioral Research Personnel created a panel to examine methods for making work force projections. It critiqued the traditional demographic projection model used by previous NRC committees and concluded that the model was unsatisfactory. Specifically, the model (1) confused "age and cohort effects" such that accurate projections could be provided only in a steady-state environment "when no projections are needed," (2) provided no means for incorporating new entrants into a field, (3) made faulty assumptions that the ratio of students to faculty and support dollars per researcher were fixed and unaffected by changing economic and technical conditions, and (4) incorrectly assumed that a current imbalance between supply and demand would not affect the future labor market (NRC, 1994, p. 21).

The NRC panel concluded that the best approaches to work force projections involved the use of "multistate period life tables." (See Appendix C for a more detailed description.) As described in the report (NRC, 1994, p. 21), such approaches

> begin by listing the characteristics of a given population (e.g., age, sector of employment, and employment status) and project changes in the population based on the life history of members of the population. . . . [Projections] are generated through a series of statistical calculations making assumptions about both the rates of transition of individuals from state to state (employed to retired, for example) and rates of new entrants to the system.

This kind of analysis can help policymakers get a sense of what the characteristics of the labor force may be in the next several years. The further out the projections go, however, the less useful they become as unforeseen events affect individual choices about educational and career options.

Unfortunately, despite the progress the present Institute of Medicine (IOM) committee made in enumerating the health services research work force, it still lacked the critical current and historical information identified above. The committee, therefore, chose not to attempt numerical projections of the size of the future health services research work force. It also did not attempt to calculate the number of new entrants that would be needed to maintain the supply of researchers at a particular level. Specifying a target work force size

---

latter average were applied to the figure for doctoral enrollment reported in the text (511), it would yield an estimated 2,700 doctoral students in the pipeline. Based on committee members' involvement in the field, this number seemed implausibly high, presumably because it would not account for attrition.

requires assumptions about the future demand for workers, a process that is even more difficult and uncertain than projecting the future supply of personnel.

Estimating the Future Demand for Personnel

Demand is conventionally described as the willingness and ability to pay for a good or service. Need is a more subjective and often more expansive concept that may be variably judged by consumers, suppliers, or "experts." Both should be considered in any discussion of future personnel requirements.

Several recent reports have expressed skepticism about "the possibility of generating useful forecasts of demand," especially long-term demand for researchers (NRC, 1994, p. 21; see also COSEPUP, 1995; and IOM, 1995). One reason is that making estimates about key factors influencing demand (e.g., funding for research, technological developments) is a highly speculative endeavor. Demand models are "sufficiently subjective and vulnerable to changing events and data limitations that they are less useful as specific numbers than as means of illuminating supply-demand dynamics" (IOM, 1995, p. 268). In addition, they do not adequately account for the behavioral responses of students, faculty, and others whose decisions about training, careers, and educational programs can shift supply away from projected levels (COSEPUP, 1995).

Even short-term indicators of demand are "of limited use to policymakers because today's decisions about fellowships and traineeships primarily affect the scientific labor market a decade from now" (NRC, 1994, p. 21). Such indicators, however, have some value because current market conditions are important influences on the career decisions young people make and because a tight current labor market might suggest different training support strategies.

Unfortunately, the health services research field lacks easily accessible information to project short-term demand. The committee's surveys of those employing health services researchers did, however, provide some qualitative perspectives on future demand as described below.

Future Prospects

Although the committee did not attempt to develop a numerical estimate of the future supply of or demand for health services researchers, it did discuss what might be expected of various factors that could affect supply or demand. These factors include (1) changes in governmental and private foundation funding for higher education and research generally and for health services research and education specifically, (2) strains on academic health centers, and (3) other restructuring of the health care system.

As this report was being drafted, prospects for federal funding for many programs and activities were highly uncertain. Even such traditionally popular programs as those for biomedical research and agricultural subsidies were being questioned. In the first proposals for reductions in expenditures for fiscal years 1996 to 2002, committees in both the U.S. Senate and the U.S. House of Representatives recommended elimination or major cutbacks in the Agency for Health Care Policy and Research, the lead agency for public funding of health services research and education (Brown, 1995).

At the state level, the committee found concerns about the willingness and ability of many states to support and maintain an ongoing program of health services research and sophisticated policy analysis. In telephone interviews, those with experience in state government cited civil service hiring restrictions, policymakers' skepticism about researchers' sensitivity to the policy considerations, and pressures on state budgets as reasons to be cautious about hiring at the state level. In addition, although health care reform initiatives may have increased demand for health services researchers (at the master's if not the doctoral level), several state reform initiatives face difficulties following the 1994 elections.

Private foundations, although not major direct employers of researchers, can be expected to continue to support health services research undertaken by academic and other organizations. Foundations, however, are also facing heavy pressure to use their resources to offset reductions in public spending for social and educational programs, and this pressure may divert some resources from research.

In many academic medical centers, economic forces and policy decisions are likely to reduce patient care income and other revenues that may have been used directly or indirectly to help support various kinds of research—including some limited amounts of health services research (Epstein, 1995). Government funding of graduate medical education and payments for services to Medicare beneficiaries are highly vulnerable to cuts. Equally serious, the relatively high costs of academic medical centers make them unattractive to managed care plans that are building provider networks. The resulting loss of patient care revenues could jeopardize the continued existence of some institutions. For other institutions, health-related research could be affected (especially in areas not of direct relevance in a competitive health care market), although cuts in external research support (e.g., government grants, industry contracts) are a greater concern.

State agencies reported that civil service rules and legislative skepticism about funding research (*analysis* is considered a more acceptable term) made employment of researchers relatively uncommon except in a few areas such as epidemiology. States tend to rely heavily on consulting firms and, sometimes, university-based consultants who can provide policy-sensitive analysis on a quick–response basis.

In business and industry, employment opportunities for health services researchers appear bright but still unpredictable in some respects. On the one hand, demand for data and analysis related to health care utilization, costs, and outcomes has been increasing as evidenced by the development of specialized firms and units to analyze organizational, clinical, and other information and to report on the performance of health care organizations.[5] On the other hand, in a competitive market, the value of research and analysis will be routinely weighed against the value of other activities in a new decisionmaking environment that is arguably less supportive of long-term investments than that which has prevailed in nonprofit environments. In addition, economic factors may well discourage the hiring of full-time workers eligible for an array of fringe benefits and other advantages, which could mean that the episodic and leaner use of outside contractors will be favored over the use of internal staff to provide research services.

The committee found consulting firms, health insurers, and similar organizations reporting that they expected to increase their hiring of master's- and doctoral-level health services researchers in the foreseeable future. Many of the employers interviewed by committee members, particularly those representing integrated health systems, pharmaceutical companies, and private consulting groups, stated they planned to double their complement of health services researchers during the next five years.

In response to the written survey's request that employers predict their recruitment plans for the next five years, more than 60 percent of responding organizations indicated that they anticipated recruiting more health services researchers in at least one of the 13 identified areas of research. Thirteen of 14 responding managed care, insurance, and similar organizations indicated they expect to recruit health services researchers in the next five years. The research areas that most respondents will recruit from are outcomes and health status measurement, health economics, biostatistics, epidemiology, and health policy analysis.

Based on respondents' reports about current recruiting difficulties and the committee's own experience, the committee expected that researchers with (1) skills in biostatistics, health economics, outcomes and health status measurement, and epidemiology, and (2) experience in managed care and research management would continue to be difficult to find for the next few years. Although the committee did not collect information on other characteristics that would make

---

[5]Interest in these organizations is sufficiently high that they are the subject of several directories, for example, yearly directories in the trade journal *Business Insurance*.

individuals more attractive in the job market, it notes the conclusion of a recent study of graduate scientists and engineers: "more employment options are available to graduate scientists and engineers who have multiple disciplines, minor degrees, personal communication skills, and entrepreneurial initiative" (COSEPUP, 1995, pp. 2–17). The implications of this discussion for training programs are considered in the next chapter.

CONCLUSION

The committee's success in achieving the study's objectives of describing the current size and characteristics of the health services research work force and projecting the future supply and demand for researchers was limited by data inadequacies. One priority became additional data collection to identify more completely the existing work force and, to a lesser extent, to gauge short–term demand for health services researchers. The resulting database of 4,920 health services researchers and information regarding demand proved illuminating, but a priority for others should be developing more complete information about the characteristics and employment patterns of the work force. Data limitations notwithstanding, the committee understood that the major factor affecting future employment will be public and private research funding. In the immediate future, the division of funding between these two major sources may shift somewhat toward the private side. As discussed in the next chapter, educational programs that prepare health services researchers will need to pay more attention to private organizations as potential employers of their students as well as potential funders of research.

4

Educational Programs, Resources, and Issues

Today's health service researchers have developed their careers through quite diverse pathways.[1] They often did not initially seek a career in health services research but migrated to the field from other areas. Such migration has sometimes—but not always—been accompanied by formal education in health services research. Researchers with doctorates from programs specifically in health services research remain relatively less common than those with discipline-based degrees, which may or may not include concentrations in health.

This chapter describes the major types of health services research educational programs and key issues or concerns about the nature and funding of education for health services research. The latter discussion pursues themes raised in Chapters 2 and 3.

---

[1]The educational paths of this committee's members (see Appendix D) illustrate this point.

EDUCATIONAL PROGRAMS

Information Sources

The most comprehensive listing of formal programs in health services research is provided by the *Directory of Training Programs in Health Services Research* compiled by the Foundation for Health Services Research (FHSR, 1992). The self-described mission of these programs is to prepare individuals to conduct health services research. If a program's primary mission is to prepare individuals for careers in management, clinical practice, or disciplinary research, it could qualify for inclusion if it provided a specific, well-defined track that prepared students to undertake health services research.

The 1991–1992 directory (the most recent) listed 121 programs in the United States and Canada, some of which offer more than one degree (e.g., both Ph.D. and M.S.). The directory includes 45 master's programs, 66 doctoral programs, and 26 fellowship programs. For each program, information is provided about its focus, structure, degree offered, size of student body and faculty, fees, and application procedures.

In early 1995, 22 programs had health services research training grants from the Agency for Health Care Policy and Research (AHCPR) under the National Research Service Award (NRSA) program (see Table 4.1). Four of these programs—three of which offered only postdoctoral work for clinicians—were not among those listed in the FHSR directory.

To better understand the current structure and capacity of health services research training programs, the committee (with funding from the Robert Wood Johnson Foundation and the Baxter Foundation) canvassed all the training programs listed in the FHSR directory. Questions dealt with such issues as program structure, focus, curriculum, student body, capacity, financial aid, and the posttraining careers of graduates. Of the 121 listed programs, 63 responded to the canvass for an overall response rate of 46 percent. (Appendix B provides more detailed information on the canvass and its limitations.)

Types of Programs

Given the number of disciplines involved in the field of health services research, counting and categorizing the programs that train health services researchers are not straightforward tasks. The diversity of the programs listed in the FHSR directory illustrates the point. Some institutions offer a formal degree in health services research. Others offer a more broadly labeled multidisciplinary degree (e.g., programs in health services management and policy). Some are clinically or professionally oriented (e.g., Ph.D. programs in nursing or social work). Other emphases within the broader field of health services research are found in M.S. and Ph.D. programs in clinical evaluative sciences and in a Ph.D. program in risk management and insurance. Many health services research programs have their organizational home in schools of public health. Several programs, particularly postdoctoral programs for clinicians, are housed in schools of medicine.

As might be expected, the 22 training programs supported by AHCPR in fiscal year (FY) 1994 (see Table 4.1) are less diverse than the 121 programs that chose to be listed in the FHSR directory. Thirteen of the AHCPR-supported programs provide both pre- and postdoctoral training in health services research; one university separately sponsors and funds both a predoctoral and a postdoctoral program. Of the seven programs offering only postdoctoral training, five limit the program to clinicians (primarily physicians).

Educational programs in health services research are differentiated by their level, focus, and depth. These characteristics relate to the degree offered, if any (e.g., M.P.H., Ph.D.), the organizational structure and disciplinary base (e.g., academic department, multidisciplinary nondepartmental program), and the amount and type of required educational work (e.g., cognate or practicum requirements, number of course hours in research methods and statistics). Student backgrounds may also differentiate programs, especially postdoctoral programs. Some programs are designed specifically for clinicians, others for Ph.D.-trained health services researchers; still others will accept additional backgrounds. (Appendix B includes a rough categorization of the FHSR-listed programs by discipline, level, and institution or program.)

Master's Degree Programs

Although "terminal" master's degree programs are common for applied fields such as health care management and public health, the basic health services research degree is clearly a doctorate. Nonetheless, graduates of general master's degree programs in health services research, health policy, public health, or related fields are an important component of the health services research work force as described in Chapters 1 and 3. Some students come to these programs with nursing, pharmacy, or other clinical degrees. Many schools offer physicians or dentists the opportunity to pursue a master's degree jointly with their clinical doctorates.

For the most part, master's programs in health services research prepare graduates to participate in research teams under the direction of more extensively

TABLE 4.1 Institutions Receiving National Research Service Awards from the Agency for Health Care Policy and Research (AHCPR), FY 1994

Program	Predoctoral	Postdoctoral
Brandeis University	X	
Brown University		X
Case Western Reserve University	X	X
Children's Hospital[a]		X
Cornell University[a]		X
Dartmouth College	X	X
Harvard University (Health Policy Program)	X	
Harvard University (School of Public Health)		X
Johns Hopkins University	X	X
New England Medical Center[a]		X
Oregon Health Sciences University/ Kaiser Permanente Center for Health Research[a]		X
Stanford University	X	X
University of California, Los Angeles/RAND Corp.	X	X
University of California, San Francisco	X	X
University of Medicine and Dentistry of New Jersey		X
University of Michigan	X	X
University of Minnesota	X	X
University of North Carolina	X	X
University of Pennsylvania	X	X
University of Rochester	X	X
University of Washington	X	X
Yale University	X	X

[a]Not listed in the 1991–1992 Foundation for Health Services Research directory of training programs.

SOURCE: Data provided to the committee by AHCPR, Division of Education, Evaluation, and Demonstrations, January 1995.

prepared investigators or to undertake applied analytic work under the direction of operational managers. Some graduates go on to doctoral work. A few become qualified principal investigators or research managers based on extensive, well-directed experience and perhaps some specialized nondoctoral training.

Doctoral Programs

Multidisciplinary programs. The committee identified a number of multidisciplinary graduate programs in health services research, although it could not determine the extent to which they were interdisciplinary (as that term is defined in Chapter 1). It is the committee's sense that the most focused, comprehensive, and intensive health services research educational programs offer a doctoral degree in health services research itself and that they use a multidisciplinary faculty, many or most of whom identify themselves as health services researchers. Doctoral programs in related areas such as public health, health management, or health policy appear to be more variable in the emphasis placed on training health services researchers as opposed to managers or policy analysts. Schools of public health often distinguish between a research-oriented Ph.D. curriculum and a D.P.H. (Doctor of Public Health) curriculum intended to develop leaders for public health services.

Disciplinary doctoral programs. Some doctoral programs in disciplines such as economics or sociology provide health-related subfields or concentrations. These disciplinary programs characteristically emphasize educational requirements in the discipline and maintain relatively few requirements within the subfield. The health services research component of a disciplinary degree may sometimes come primarily through dissertation or other research experience. Disciplinary programs often rely on schools of public health or other health-related programs located elsewhere in their parent university to provide coursework and faculty supervision for their health services research subfield. Courses in health economics, medical sociology, or health policy may also be taught in economics, sociology, or political science departments.

Postdoctoral Programs

Programs for clinicians. Some postdoctoral programs are designed specifically to provide clinicians (those who already have M.D.s or other clinical degrees) with training in health services research methods. For example, one track in Dartmouth's program in evaluative clinical sciences "is focused on individuals who will combine clinical residencies with education and research in

. . . an integrated program that adds one year to the residency and results in a [Master of Science degree]" (FHSR, 1992, p. 12). (Dartmouth also has a Ph.D. program targeted at physicians.) There is at least one postdoctoral fellowship in health services research specifically for dentists, and several universities and Department of Veterans Affairs (VA) medical centers offer master's degrees or postdoctoral health services research programs for physicians. Such programs attract many young clinicians, but they also provide a significant opportunity for midcareer change.

Other postdoctoral programs. Other postdoctoral programs provide an opportunity for those with recent doctorates in health services research and related fields to concentrate on specific research interests and to develop experience that will increase their likelihood of securing research funding. These postdoctoral experiences generally do not lead to an additional degree. In addition to university sites, postdoctoral programs may be offered by nonacademic organizations such as hospitals and managed care organizations. The latter may offer academically oriented researchers an opportunity to move into more applied kinds of research and research management.

On-the-Job Training and Continuing Education

A variety of programs and activities aim to extend the knowledge and skills of those already in the health work force. Many individuals who are already educated in one or another basic discipline receive training and education in health services research through structured short courses or seminars that provide instruction in specific topics, such as outcomes measurement and the use of analytic software packages. On-the-job education may take the form of mentoring, which can guide the development and maturation of newly graduated health services researchers. More generally, work itself is a critical educational experience.

In addition, reflecting a recent trend, many health services research education programs are reconsidering the traditional, full-time, residential format and offering options that better accommodate students who want to continue to work or enroll on a part-time basis. Classes are now being offered during evenings and weekends and through distance learning arrangements (e.g., mail, video). Several programs are specifically designed for business and government executives or midcareer professionals who want training in health services research. To meet the need for lifelong learning and career flexibility, university programs, professional groups, and other organizations also offer training through a variety of means, including short courses and summer institutes.

Current Program Enrollments

As described in Chapter 3's discussion of the research work force pipeline, the committee estimated that the health services research programs enroll at least 1,015 students in master's programs, 511 in doctoral programs, and another 197 in postdoctoral fellowship programs. (Appendix B notes why limitations in enrollment data make it likely that this estimate is low.) As was true for the health services research work force in general, the committee was not able to categorize participants in health services research training programs by gender or ethnicity.

Based on its experience but no directly relevant data, the committee thought the problem of underrepresentation in educational programs was more of a concern for minorities than for women (although the latter may be underrepresented in various segments of the work force). The committee sees no reason to expect that African-American, Hispanic, and other minorities who are generally underrepresented in advanced education would be found in health services research programs in numbers proportional to their share of the population. Health services research programs probably compete with medical, dental, and other professional schools for the relatively limited pool of minority college graduates, a problem noted in other reports on advanced education in the health professions and in science and engineering (NRC, 1994, IOM, 1994a). These reports have argued that efforts to increase minority representation must focus on broadening the educational pipeline at the precollegiate level (see, for example, University of California, 1993; IOM, 1994a, 1995). Strategies for achieving this objective generally call for cooperation among educational institutions, governments, corporations, and private foundations in developing college and career information resources, curriculum guidance and support programs for schools, mentoring programs for individual students, and similar activities. At the undergraduate and graduate levels, affordable tuition and financial assistance are important, as is a supportive learning environment.

Curricula and Preparation for the "Real World"

Core Courses

No accrediting or other standard-setting organization provides curriculum guidelines for health services research programs, and federal awards for training programs do not have explicit curriculum prescriptions. Moreover, because educational programs in health services research vary in level, focus, and objectives, their curricula necessarily vary. Doctoral programs, for instance, will generally provide more coursework in research methods and statistics than master's programs. Programs in disciplines such as economics typically emphasize discipline-specific courses over health-related topics.

Certain courses, however, tend to be viewed as the core of a health services research curriculum. Although the only course cited by a majority of survey respondents for all program levels (master's, doctoral, and fellowship) was research methods, majorities or near-majorities also cited statistics or biostatistics (see Table B.4 in Appendix B). Health economics was another quantitatively oriented course cited by more than one-third of respondents in each program area. Given the committee's own judgments as well as what it learned about the demand for researcher capabilities, it agreed that these areas should generally be part of the core curriculum. The committee noted with some concern that health care organization was mentioned as a core course by less than one-third of respondents in each of the program areas, although larger proportions mentioned health policy, a subject that may have considerable overlap with health care organization. Whatever the label, the committee viewed a solid understanding of the health care system as an essential part of education in health services research.

Preparation for the "Real World"

In addition to standard coursework, it is valuable for students to be involved in ongoing health services research under the supervision of a mentor. Ideally, students should be exposed to all phases of research—from initial development of the project to final dissemination of the findings. Practical experience in proposal writing and fund raising is also valuable. Students who plan a career in academia should, in particular, be encouraged to write articles for scholarly journals and to present academic papers at professional conferences. Students who want to be prepared for careers in government or the private sector should be directed to internships or similar experiences that will expose them to the particular demands and stresses of research and policy analyses in these settings. Stresses include the need for quick turnaround of analyses, writing styles that are less academic, rapid shifts in target issues, and sensitivity to client needs and demands. In government, researchers may find that seriously incomplete or flawed analyses (e.g., unadjusted studies of hospital mortality data) are made public prematurely, whereas researchers in managed care or insurance organizations may chafe under proprietary restrictions on publication of their analyses.

Another part of the real world of health services research that most students will face is participating in studies as a member of a research or project team. Given the multidisciplinary nature of the field and the variety of educational paths that lead there, researchers will often find themselves working with individuals from varied disciplinary or clinical backgrounds and different levels of training and experience. As this study proceeded, the committee became concerned that those in doctoral programs are not routinely educated to value the contributions of master's level researchers, to understand what may reasonably be expected from other researchers and from clinicians, or to develop the qualities needed to lead or participate effectively in a research team. Such qualities include communication skills, facility in group decisionmaking processes, and knowledge of conflict resolution strategies. For work in many industry settings, effective participation in project teams may also require skills in understanding client needs and crafting analyses that are both methodologically sound and acceptable, persuasive, and even attractive to clients. In the governmental world, a similar appreciation is needed for the expectations of policymakers in the administrative and legislative branches.

Students will vary in the degree to which they are temperamentally suited for academic, industry, governmental, or other settings, and schooling cannot substitute for the learning that occurs in a real job in industry or government. Educational programs can, nonetheless, help students to understand and cultivate the intellectual and personal qualities needed to succeed in a variety of environments.

Given recent trends in employment, it is the general sense of the committee that health services research programs will benefit their students by providing broader rather than narrower educational opportunities. These include opportunities for coursework in several disciplines and methodological techniques, practical experience in research and policy analysis, development of skills in teamwork and communication, and exposure to differences in expectations for researchers held by academic, government, and industry employers. Health services researchers have versatile and marketable skills in such areas as conducting oral interviews and focus groups, locating information sources, interpreting published reports and data, and synthesizing information. For those considering a career shift, for example, from academic to industry employment, special continuing education programs may be useful in building or refreshing the knowledge or skill base needed for such a shift.

FUNDING FOR EDUCATION IN HEALTH SERVICES RESEARCH

Support for training in health services research comes in several forms and from a variety of sources. The federal government and other organizations provide some grants to students directly but also provide grants to institutional programs, which, in turn, support students. Students themselves contribute through tuition payments, and state taxpayers help support programs in public institutions. Research grants that include research assistantships serve the joint purpose of supporting research and training. Teaching assistantships likewise serve a dual purpose. Foundations and corporations may provide special-purpose grants or gifts for purposes such as curriculum development or endowed professorships.

Federal Programs

The federal government provides the majority of dedicated funding for health services research education. A key vehicle for this support is the NRSA program, which provides grants to educational institutions (which make traineeship awards to individual pre- and postdoctoral students) and to individuals directly in the form of fellowships. Other, more indirect mechanisms support some training, including federal research grants that fund research assistantships for students and awards for dissertation research.

Historical Context

As described in Chapter 2, the federal government funded some health services research before the 1960s.[2] The first formal support specifically for training in the field, however, awaited the 1967 decision establishing the National Center for Health Services Research and Development (NCHSR). NCHSR's Health Services Training Grants program provided awards to qualified public or private institutions for education programs to educate "competent investigators in the methods and techniques of conducting health services research including analysis, development and demonstration projects" (USDHEW, 1970, p. 1). Institutions could focus on the organization, delivery, quality, financing, utilization, and evaluation of health services delivery systems. Program grants included funds for institutional expenses as well as stipends for trainees. In 1970, stipends ranged from $3,000 to $4,700 ($11,575 to $18,134 in 1994 dollars), depending on an individual's work and educational experience, and other trainee expenses including tuition might also be covered. The program accounted for about 8 percent of NCHSR's appropriations for the years 1968 to 1973 (undated, unpublished document from DHHS files, about 1983).

In 1972, the report *Improving Health Care through Research and Development* noted "constant pressure [on NCHSR] to curtail research training

---

[2]Congress first granted the Public Health Service authority to train health researchers in 1930 in the Ransdell Act (P.L. 71-251), which created the National Institutes of Health (NIH) and provided for research fellowships at the NIH and other medical or research centers. When the National Cancer Institute was created in 1937, it had legislative instructions to create what became a formal fellowship program (NRC, 1975a, 1994). As subsequent institutes were created, the training authority was expanded.

programs" (PSAC, 1972, p. 3). Shortly afterwards, the Nixon administration recommended phasing out most of the health training programs for biomedical, clinical, and other health researchers on the grounds that the programs were unnecessary and were inefficient in generating researchers (NRC, 1979). Following considerable debate, Congress responded in 1974 with the National Research Service Award Act (P.L. 93-348). The legislation consolidated and restructured programs in the various institutes of the NIH. It also called for continuing study of training needs and asked the National Academy of Sciences to undertake this activity and make recommendations for "serious legislative consideration." The National Research Council (NRC) issued its first report on personnel needs and training for biomedical and behavioral research in 1975 and its most recent report in 1994. (See NRC, 1994, for a historical review.)

The 1974 legislation did not affect clinical training, nor did it affect "authority available elsewhere in the Public Health Service Act under which the Secretary may enter into contracts with public and private entities and individuals for health services research and health statistics training" (NRC, 1975b, p. 1). For FY 1974, however, the Office of Management and Budget (OMB) refused to allow NCHSR to use any appropriated funds for training programs after existing trainees and fellows completed their terms (NRC, 1976). All NCHSR support ceased in FY 1976, although the Alcohol, Drug Abuse, and Mental Health Administration (ADAMHA) continued NRSA awards in health services research. In 1980, ADAMHA reclassified its awards so that the disciplines or fields (e.g., public health, economics, and psychology) covered by the health services research category were reclassified as either behavioral or clinical sciences awards (NRC, 1981).

During the 1970s and 1980s, various NRC and Institute of Medicine (IOM) committees repeatedly recommended reestablishment of the health services research training program. The 1979 report, for example, stated that health services research was a national need, and it emphasized the importance of federal support for health services research training (NRC, 1979). The reports also continued to include recommendations for numbers of health services research training awards.

Nonetheless, OMB continued to refuse departmental requests to support health services research training, even after the Health Services Research, Health Statistics, and Medical Technology Act of 1978 (P.L. 95-623) explicitly authorized the extension of NRSA to cover health services research training. Through the early 1980s, NCHSR provided only minor and somewhat indirect training support that covered a few research fellows in the agency's intramural research program (which were equivalent to postdoctoral fellowships for new or established researchers), an unknown number of research assistants (as part of project grants), and several dissertation research awards.

Table 4.2 presents the number of trainee positions funded and fellowships awarded in health services research by the NCHSR and the AHCPR from 1967 to 1994.[3] Table 4.3 presents the recommendations for health services research traineeships and fellowships made by the NRC or the IOM from 1976 to 1994. The actual and recommended numbers of awards have consistently been far apart, most notably, of course, during the years when no awards were made.

In 1986, NRSA awards in health services research were finally reinstituted. At that time, NIH allocated 0.5 percent of its total NRSA budget (or approximately $1.1 million) for health services research. The awards were administered by NCHSR and later by AHCPR after it was created in 1989 (replacing NCHSR). AHCPR decided to supplement the NRSA allocation it received from NIH; from FY 1990 through 1992, more than one-third of total health services research NRSA funds came from AHCPR internal funds. The NIH Revitalization Act of 1993 increased the NIH allotment for health services research to 1 percent of the total NRSA budget (about $3.5 million in FY 1993). Despite this increase in funding, AHCPR has continued to supplement the NIH allocation. Table 4.4 and Figure 4.1 summarize funding for the NRSA health services research awards since FY 1986.

Current NRSA Program

Today, NRSA awards (institutional pre- and postdoctoral traineeships and individual postdoctoral fellowships) provide one of the most important resources to individuals wishing to pursue predoctoral or postdoctoral training in health services research. Although AHCPR makes most of these awards, the National Institute of Mental Health supports training in mental health services research.[4] Given the multidisciplinary, and hence nondepartmental, nature of health services research, NRSA institutional awards provide important support to institutions working to develop such broad-based programs.

---

[3] NRSA awards from some NIH institutes, including the National Institute of Alcohol Abuse and Alcoholism, the National Institute on Drug Abuse, and the National Institute of Mental Health, also support the training of health services researchers as well as clinical and basic science researchers. However, because the institutes do not classify their awards as health services research, the number of awardees receiving training in health services research through these agencies cannot be determined.

[4] As noted in Chapter 2, the National Institute of Nursing Research does not have health services research as part of its explicit research and training mandate, but many of its NRSA awards support students training in health services research as defined in this report.

TABLE 4.2 Awards for Health Services Research Training, 1967–1994

Fiscal Year of Award	Institutional Grants	Number of Traineeships	Number of Fellowships	Total
1967	15	85	22	107
1968	16	105	31	136
1969	21	152	32	184
1970	50	267	61	328
1971	51	330	82	412
1972	49	347	90	437
1973	44	327	50	377
1974	40	348	35[a]	383
1975	36	212[a]	11	223
1976 (est.)	20	110	4	114
No Awards Were Granted 1977–1985				
1986	7	33	7	40
1987	8	39	7	46
1988	8	40	6	46
1989	10	36	7	43
1990	10	73	14	87
1991	11	65	12	77
1992	13	92	12	104
1993	16	95	17	112
1994	22	114	19	133

NOTE: Awards given during the period FY 1969–1989 were from the National Center for Health Services Research; those for FY 1990–1994 were from the Agency for Health Care Policy and Research (AHCPR).

[a]No new fellowships were awarded after FY 1973 and no training grants after FY 1974; the numbers shown for 1975 and 1976 represent continuing commitments.

SOURCE: Compiled from NRC, 1976, 1979, 1981, and 1994, and from data provided to the committee by AHCPR, Division of Education, Evaluation, and Demonstration, July 1995.

TABLE 4.3 Recommendations for National Research Service Awards for Health Services Research by Committees of the National Research Council (NRC) or the Institute of Medicine (IOM), 1976–1994

Report	Years Covered by Recommendations	Year 1	Year 2	Year 3
1976 NRC[a]	1976, 1977, 1978	185	185	185
1977 NRC[b]	1979, 1980, 1981	250 300	275 440	300 440
1978 NRC[a]	1981, 1982, 1983	275	300	330
1979 NRC[a]	(explicitly reiterated 1978 recommendations)			
1981 NRC[a]	1982, 1983, 1984	330	330	330
1983 IOM[c]	1985, 1986, 1987	330	330	330
1985 IOM[c]	1988, 1989, 1990	330	330	330
1989 NRC[c]	(reiterated 1985 recommendations)			
1994 NRC[d]	1994, 1995, 1996–1999	115	240	360[e]

[a] This recommendation is for Alcohol, Drug Abuse, and Mental Health Administration (ADAMHA) slots only.
[b] The committee made specific recommendations for both ADAMHA (top number) and National Center for Health Services Research (NCHSR) (bottom number) slots.
[c] This recommendation is for both ADAMHA and NCHSR slots; no allocation between the two agencies was given.
[d] This recommendation is for AHCPR slots only.
[e] The committee also recommended 360 awards each year for 1996–1999.

SOURCES: NRC, 1976, 1977, 1978, 1979, 1981, 1989, 1994; IOM, 1983, 1985.

TABLE 4.4 Funding of National Research Service Awards (NRSA) for Health Services Research, FY 1986–1994

Fiscal Year	Total NRSA Expenditure
1986	$1,146,379
1987	1,274,000
1988	1,308,136
1989	1,322,975
1990	2,588,749[a]
1991	2,500,832[a]
1992	3,141,342[a]
1993	3,645,090[a]
1994	4,310,662[a]

NOTE: From FY 1986 through FY 1992, the Agency for Health Care Policy and Research (AHCPR) received 0.5 percent of the total NRSA assessment appropriated to the National Institutes of Health (NIH). Beginning FY 1993, AHCPR's assessment from NIH increased from 0.5 percent to 1 percent of the total NIH NRSA appropriation.

[a]Totals for these years included supplementary funds from AHCPR (See Figure 4.1).

SOURCE: Data provided to the committee by AHCPR, Division of Education, Evaluation, and Demonstrations, January 1995.

Table 4.5 describes some of the key features of both the institutional and individual NRSA grants. Essentially, both types of awards provide for student stipends and a limited amount of money to defray some expenses of training and to cover trainee's expenses for medical insurance and some travel to scientific meetings.

Although NRSA stipends are not considered salaries and are not subject to any costs normally associated with employee benefits (such as deductions for FICA, workers' compensation, or unemployment taxes), the stipend is counted and taxed as part of the student's gross income. Postdoctoral (but not predoctoral) trainees and fellows are required to pay back their awards. They may do so by making a cash payment or by performing health services research or teaching on the basis of roughly one month of service for every month of the

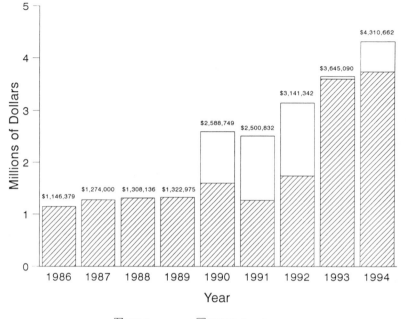

Figure 4.1 Funding for National Research Service Awards in health service research, FY 1986 through 1994. SOURCE: Data provided to the committee by the Agency for Health Care Policy and Research (AHCPR), Division of Education, Evaluation, and Demonstrations, January 1995.

first 12 months of postdoctoral NRSA support they receive. Because the fellows can count their second year of NRSA-supported activity towards their payback requirement, those who have completed a two-year fellowship are considered to have fulfilled their payback obligations.

Institutional pre- and postdoctoral traineeships. In FY 1994, the AHCPR awarded training grants to 22 institutions to develop or enhance research training opportunities for individuals interested in health services research. These awards assist health services research programs to develop multi- and interdisciplinary curricula, faculty, and research activities. As described earlier, the programs may provide both pre- and postdoctoral training or both. Some programs are targeted solely to preparing clinicians in health services research. In addition to university-based programs, awards may go to other institutions (e.g., Children's Hospital in Boston).

TABLE 4.5 Key Features of National Research Service Awards Traineeships and Fellowships

Feature	Traineeships	Fellowships
Stipend Predoctoral	$10,008	NA
Postdoctoral	(Same schedule used for both trainees and fellows)	

Years of Postdoctoral Experience	Stipend ($)
Less than 1	19,608
1	20,700
2	25,600
3	26,900
4	28,200
5	29,500
6	30,800
7 or more	32,300

Feature	Traineeships	Fellowships
Indirect costs	Equal to 8% of the institution's total allowable direct costs or the institution's actual indirect cost rate, whichever is less.	None
Trainee tuition, fees, travel, and health insurance	Can be reimbursed	NA
Other training costs	$1,500 per predoctoral trainee	$3,000 per fellow (Fellows at for profit institutions receive only $2,000.)
	$2,500 per postdoctoral trainee	

NA = not applicable.

SOURCES: AHCPR, 1994a, b.

NRSA grants to institutions from AHCPR totaled more than $3.7 million in FY 1994. The grants ranged from $69,272 to $289,999 and funded between 2 and 10 trainees at each institution. In total, 114 individuals received support through the program. The committee heard suggestions that current institutional awards cover a smaller proportion of institutional costs than in the early 1970s. For example, awards in the earlier period included significant salary support for program directors. Detailed information was not, however, readily available to allow specific comparisons between current and past awards.

Predoctoral trainees at all levels of experience received an annual stipend of $10,008. (Stipends for postdoctoral trainees follow the same schedule as postdoctoral fellowships, which are described in the next section.) In 1994, the NRC recommended that predoctoral stipends be increased to approximately $12,000 for FY 1996. As mentioned earlier, the $3,000 to $4,700 stipends of the early 1970s would be worth $11,575 to $18,134 when adjusted for inflation. The early stipends were not taxed, but current awards are subject to income taxes. Thus, current stipends are demonstrably less generous than in previous years.

Individual postdoctoral fellowships. Unlike the institutional grants, NRSA postdoctoral fellowships are awarded directly to individuals. Applications are accepted three times a year: December, April, and August. Those fellowships may be particularly helpful to women or other students who might not have as much flexibility to relocate to enroll at a NRSA-designated institution.

Nineteen individuals received postdoctoral fellowships from AHCPR in FY 1994. Their stipends were based on the same scale as is used for the institutional traineeships. The fellows' stipends for the first year of support were determined by the number of full years of relevant postdoctoral experience at the time of the appointment. Stipends ranged from $19,608 for those with less than one year of postdoctoral experience to $32,300 for those with seven or more years of relevant experience. Institutions may (and frequently do) supplement these stipends.

Institutions offering postdoctoral fellowship positions typically receive no NRSA payments and must cover all their costs through research grants or other sources, which creates some problems. In basic science research, postdoctoral fellows tend to fit readily into their mentors' laboratories and can begin immediately to carry out part of their mentors' basic programs of research. In health services research, although the fellows may become a part of their mentors' overall research teams, mentors may find it more difficult to segment parts of complex health services research projects in ways that allow fellows to produce short- and intermediate-term payoffs. Moreover, because fellows are not usually enrolled students, they do not pay tuition, nor are they routinely considered part of a department or a faculty member's teaching load. Without these kinds of institutional support from ACHPR or the university, department or faculty members may incur substantial costs for their mentoring activities. Some of the best investigators may, as a result, be reluctant to accept additional postdoctoral students.

Other Federal Programs

The federal government also supports health services research educational programs by awarding grants in support of dissertation research. AHCPR has awarded such grants since 1975. In FY 1994, 23 students received grants of up to $20,000 to support their dissertation research in health services. Students apply for the grants in January and awards are announced in the summer. The Health Care Financing Administration also provides health services research dissertation grants, although their grants are applied for in October and awarded by December.

The VA, through its Academic Affairs and Health Services Research and Development offices, conducts and supports pre- and postdoctoral training programs at 13 VA medical centers. Since 1983, the program has trained 113 predoctoral students and 38 postdoctoral students in health services research. An additional 78 physicians received technical assistance or training in health services research during their VA-supported postdoctoral fellowships in such fields as ambulatory care, geropsychology, and women's health. The stipends given to these students and fellows are somewhat higher than NRSA awards. Predoctoral students receive between $15,700 and $17,000 a year, postdoctoral students receive $34,000 a year, and physicians' stipends are indexed to match their salaries at an affiliated school of medicine.

Nonfederal Programs

A significant source of support for health services research training comes from the educational programs themselves. Many universities award scholarships, waive tuition and fees, and provide teaching assistantships and other employment opportunities to their students. Even if a program receives federal funds (NRSA or other), those funds often must be supplemented with internal monies in order to provide the competitive stipend and benefit package that will attract top students. Several state governments directly and indirectly support health services research education by subsidizing the programs offered through their state universities and by providing some grants for research and, less commonly, training.

Some foundations and private companies also offer training support to health services researchers, although support more often comes indirectly through grants for research. Formal training support from private industry has typically been given to students in specific areas, such as pharmacoeconomics or managed care administration, rather than to students in more general health services research programs. Some private organizations sponsor students on semester or year-long internships to expose them to how health services research is carried out in the for-profit environment. For example, U.S. Quality Algorithms (a subsidiary of U.S. Healthcare) is sponsoring a one-year managed care fellowship at the medical college of Thomas Jefferson University in Philadelphia. Another way for industry to support health services research educational programs is through the endowment of faculty chairs; Blue Cross of California recently did this by endowing a chair in health care financing at the University of Southern California.

The Pew Charitable Trusts has long sponsored innovative educational programs in health services research through its Health Policy Program. The Pew program enables current and future leaders in health care to pursue doctorate and postdoctorate training in health policy at three sites: Brandeis University, the University of Michigan, and the University of California, San Francisco (UCSF). Each of the three programs has developed a unique educational model. Brandeis University offers a two-year accelerated, interdisciplinary program leading to a Ph.D. in health policy. The University of Michigan runs a three-year intensive, nonresidential program designed so that students can remain employed full time while obtaining a doctorate in public health. The UCSF program provides one- or two-year postdoctoral fellowships to social scientists, physicians, and other health professionals.

The Robert Wood Johnson Foundation also supports education in health services research through its Scholars in Health Policy Research Program, which offers two-year postdoctoral training to recent graduates in economics, political science, and sociology to advance their involvement in health policy research. The foundation also sponsors the Clinical Scholars Program, which provides postdoctoral fellowships specifically for young physicians to help them develop research skills in nonbiological disciplines that are relevant to medical care.

CONCLUSION

Formal education or training in health services research takes many different forms that draw students from different programs and prepare them for varied roles and careers. Programs range from the master's to the postdoctoral level. Short courses, summer institutes, and other opportunities add further diversity. Health services research may be the principal focus of a multidisciplinary educational program or a secondary emphasis in a disciplinary or professional program. Although the committee stressed the importance of doctoral programs devoted to health services research, other program models are also valid.

The committee noted that funding for education in health services research has been unstable and generally limited. Although funding has increased in recent years, it is still below levels achieved in the early 1970s. The next chapter summarizes the committee's findings and presents its recommendations.

5

Findings and Recommendations

In a health care system undergoing rapid and complex change, the challenges for health services researchers are imposing. The pace of change, the multiplicity of involved parties, and the limited availability of crucial data make it difficult to describe what is happening, much less explain it or track the consequences. In the policy arena, budgetary constraints and, in some cases, skepticism about research may impede investigations that could guide the change or identify its unwanted consequences. Another potential problem is a lack of appropriately educated health services researchers.

This chapter presents the committee's findings and recommendations on health services research work force and training issues. These conclusions respond to the request from the Agency for Health Care Policy and Research (AHCPR) for assessments of the current and future work force and for recommendations to inform decisions about federal resources for educating health services researchers. The conclusions and recommendations are also intended to be useful to other government agencies (e.g., the Department of Veterans Affairs), educators, and private organizations, including foundations and employers that support health services research or education.

DATA AVAILABILITY AND IMPROVEMENT

One of the committee's first findings was that existing data on the size and characteristics of the health services research work force are fragmentary. The committee sought and obtained private funding to collect additional information from a variety of sources, including employers. The resulting database is the most extensive available listing of the health services research work force, but it still lacks important information about the characteristics of those listed.

The committee urges the Association for Health Services Research (AHSR) to seek funding to update and extend the database through a more detailed survey of researcher characteristics including, for example, age, gender, ethnicity, and employment status. In addition, the committee encourages the National Science Foundation and the National Research Council (NRC) to consider revising the annual census of those who have received doctorates and the longitudinal sample survey of doctoral recipients to allow better identification of those educated or working in the field of health services research. Such steps would provide information useful for understanding the dynamics of the health services research work force. Finally, as part of a more general government effort to evaluate the results of various research training programs, the committee recommends that the AHCPR and other relevant government agencies investigate the career paths and productivity of trainee and fellowship recipients.

These recommendations are consistent with those of a recent report on graduate scientists and engineers (COSEPUP, 1995). That report's main recommendation was that "the National Science Foundation and the National Research Council should continue to improve the coverage, timeliness and analysis of data on the education and employment of scientists and engineers to support better national decision-making about human resources in science and technology" (pp. 5–14). A more specific recommendation was for an increase in information on nonacademic employment to reflect the increasing importance of employment in this sector.

WORK FORCE SIZE AND CHARACTERISTICS

The committee identified approximately 5,000 current health services researchers. This estimate undoubtedly omits some health services researchers and includes some individuals who are interested in health services research but not actually engaged in it.

Approximately 50 percent of the researchers for whom degree information was available have doctoral degrees, and another 28 percent (mostly physicians) have clinical degrees. The proportion of the work force whose doctorates are specifically in health services research rather than another field or discipline could not be determined. Given the number, size, and age of programs offering degrees in health services research or closely related fields (primarily health policy or health care management), however, the committee believes it likely that only a minority of researchers now have such degrees.

The largest segments of the current health services research work force appear to be employed in academic institutions and private research organizations and consulting groups. Employment in health plans, insurance companies, and similar organizations appears to have been growing fast, albeit from a smaller base. As noted in Chapter 3, a recent study indicates that for graduate scientists and engineers in general, academic jobs are declining while positions in business and industry are growing.

Without information on researchers' age, employment history, or percentage of time spent in research, life table models or other work force estimation methods cannot be employed to arrive at reasonable numerical projections of the future supply of health services researchers. On qualitative grounds, however, the committee foresees growth in the health services research work force *if* public research funding escapes significant reductions and *if* competitors in the emerging health care market continue to support growth in knowledge about the quality, effectiveness, and cost of clinical services, the behavioral determinants of health status, and similar questions.

SUPPLY IN RELATION TO DEMAND

Current Supply and Demand

The committee was not able to make an empirically based, quantitative statement about the match between current supply and current demand for health services researchers. In particular, it was unable to find systematic data on underemployment and unemployment levels for researchers or on other variables that would support such a statement.

However, based on interviews with health services research employers and on the experience of committee members, the committee reached two qualitative conclusions. First, no anecdotal or other evidence suggests that the current supply of health services researchers exceeds current demand. Second, employers appear to be more concerned about the quality than the quantity of prospective researchers. Well-trained researchers with practical experience in health care organizations (e.g., integrated health care systems, insurance companies) and experience in managing research units appear to be in short supply. Recruiting difficulties also appear to exist for those trained in both health services research and selected disciplinary areas including statistics, epidemiology, health economics, and outcomes and health status measurement. In some clinical areas, such as oral health and allied health services, trained health services researchers also appear to be scarce.

Future Supply and Demand

The committee identified several factors that may affect the future supply of and demand for health services researchers, although economic, technological, political, and other uncertainties make specific predictions risky. On the need or potential demand side, this report has identified many major questions for health services research, and it has underscored the importance of understanding the nature and effects of rapid changes in the health care system. For the foreseeable future, the committee expects that demand for health services researchers with particular degrees or skills will reflect the increased emphasis that public and private decisionmakers are placing on market forces (and therefore informed consumer choice of health plans and care options) in the health care sector. That is, demand will continue for researchers prepared to build knowledge about health outcomes, health status measurement, quality assessment, patient and consumer decisionmaking, informatics, and related areas.

The prospects for some employment sectors are uncertain, particularly those dependent on government funding. For academic institutions, where most researchers are now employed, relative or absolute contractions in funding for education and research from federal and state governments are anticipated by many policy analysts and educators. In a financially stressed university environment, the multidisciplinary character of programs in health services research (and research education) may leave such programs more vulnerable to reduction or elimination than longer-established and more easily defined programs in specific disciplines. This vulnerability may be offset, to some degree, if health services research programs can document growth in the applicant pool, employer demand for graduates, and financial support for students from actual or potential employers through mechanisms such as tuition reimbursements and research funding.

In addition, most academic health centers are facing declines in patient care revenues as health care plans bypass these centers in favor of institutions that are less specialized, less comprehensive, less involved in health-related training and research of any kind, and thereby less costly. Overall, the demand and economic rewards for most categories of specialty and subspecialty clinicians appear likely to decline, and surpluses are anticipated. As a result, some additional physicians, nurses, and other clinicians may seek education and employment in health services research.

TRAINING PROGRAMS

The committee encourages continued evolution of formal educational programs in health services research. These programs play a special role by providing (1) an organizing focus for the field, (2) an environment supportive of creative research and methodology development, and (3) an important source of personnel prepared to increase the knowledge base for responding to issues of cost, quality, and access facing the nation. The committee believes that they encourage systematic, multidisciplinary investigation and understanding of health services, behaviors, and outcomes and, further, that they promote the formulation of research frameworks and strategies that integrate the theories, concepts, and tools of different disciplines. They are, therefore, a valuable national resource.

Still, a single educational path is neither practical nor desirable. Health services research will continue to attract and benefit from people with a variety of disciplinary and clinical degrees who are prepared to make important theoretical, conceptual, and empirical contributions to the field. To take full advantage of this variety, the field needs to provide a range of training opportunities for those who are pursuing or have completed graduate degrees in other areas. It is, however, desirable and important for these researchers also to have explicit training in health services research through either a disciplinary or, ideally, a multidisciplinary program.

To the extent that recruiting problems exist in some discipline or skill areas, employers may resort to on-the-job training and short-term programs. The committee believes that such limited training is not, in general, sufficient preparation for those who are expected to design and conduct high-quality health services research. Some formal academic training is important.

Academic training is only a partial answer for the experience-related areas of apparent shortage, particularly in areas such as managed care or research management where on-the-job training and seasoning yield essential background. Worksite-based internships and fellowships may also help to bridge the gap between the university and the workplace.

These findings led the committee to recommend some shifts in the focus of publicly supported training in health services research. In particular, the committee recommended that AHCPR

• consider greater emphasis for some predoctoral and postdoctoral awards on training in areas such as outcomes and health status measurement, biostatistics, epidemiology, health economics, and health policy in which recruiting difficulties have been reported;

• more explicitly consider—in evaluating institutional training program awards—how an applicant's training approach, faculty, research opportunities, and training slots relate to personnel shortage areas; and

• set aside a substantial percentage of institutional awards for innovative programs in health services research, which might be completely new programs or significant modifications of existing programs (see below).

The committee offered no ranked prescription for the program innovations to be encouraged. By way of example, however, innovative programs might be designed to

- explore new models and methods for truly multidisciplinary and interdisciplinary education and investigation;
- test creative educational opportunities and technologies for midcareer professionals with varied levels and kinds of educational backgrounds and work experiences;
- extend student and faculty research experiences in nonacademic settings through mechanisms such as internships and faculty sabbaticals;
- develop strategies to involve more community-based practitioners in outcomes and related research originated and managed by faculty investigators; or
- cultivate partnerships with public or private organizations to encourage collaborative research training, joint methodology development, or other cooperative ventures.

Several of these examples point toward educational programs that are more community and customer oriented, that is, that prepare students better for employment in government and industry as well as academic settings. Such innovative steps may be somewhat more costly than current programs. AHCPR should consider providing some additional funds to cover better the institutional costs of developing innovative educational experiences.

The committee also felt that greater flexibility in the timing of dissertation grant awards was desirable to better accommodate students' schedules. It therefore recommends that the agencies awarding such grants, including AHCPR and the Health Care Financing Administration, offer multiple award cycles throughout the year instead of the current once-a-year cycle. The committee also noted the problems of nontraditional students, including single parents and others with significant family responsibilities. Most predoctoral programs require people to be in residence for one to two years, although a few provide on-the-job or on-campus options that provide greater flexibility. Flexibility in postdoctoral programs also warrants consideration.

The committee endorsed the recommendations for health services research training awards that were issued in 1994 by the NRC Committee on National Needs for Biomedical and Behavioral Research Personnel. The recommendations called for 360 National Research Service Awards (NRSA) yearly for fiscal years 1996 through 1999. This recommendation was up slightly from the 330 NRSA awards recommended in several reports during the 1970s and 1980s. It would still leave the number of awards at a slightly lower level than prevailed for health services research in the early 1970s but would more than double the actual 1994 numbers.

The committee also supported three other NRC recommendations for the NRSA program that focused on stipends and on women and underrepresented minorities. The recommendations called for the program to

1. "raise the real value of stipends to more competitive levels by fiscal 1996: approximately $12,000 per year for predoctoral awardees and approximately $25,000 for postdoctoral awardees with less than 2 years of research experience [and] maintain the real value of these stipends (i.e., the nominal value adjusted for inflation) through annual increases of 3 percent per year (the assumed annual rate of inflation)" (NRC, 1994, p. 2);

2. "examine research training opportunities for women through the NRSA program and strengthen the role of postdoctoral support to assist women in establishing themselves in productive careers as research scientists" (NRC, 1994, p. 8); and

3. "hold Minority Access to Research Careers (MARC) awards constant at fiscal 1993 levels, or approximately 680 awards, pending the outcome of . . . [a not-yet-published] NIH evaluation study" (NRC, 1994, p. 8).

CONCLUSION

As this report was being drafted, events were unfolding that promised to be quite significant for the health services research work force and related educational programs. Specifically, a quite dramatic market-driven restructuring of the health care system was well under way, one that could significantly disrupt established patterns of patient care and relationships between clinicians and patients and affect the cost, availability, and quality of health care.

Restructuring is likely to bring both positive and negative effects and to distribute benefits and burdens unequally across different income, age, and other population groups. The committee believes it critical that the nation sustain the research capacity—including funding, personnel, and educational programs—to document and understand these changes and their consequences.

Recently, however, some in Congress were calling for the elimination of AHCPR as a cost-cutting measure (Brown, 1995). In the context of market-oriented strategies for containing health care costs, abolition or near elimination of AHCPR and its focused health services research and training agenda could undermine the development of knowledge important for effectively functioning and accountable markets and for assessing the impact of health care restructuring on the public's health and, especially, on the availability and quality of care for the nation's most vulnerable children and adults.

Although an array of private organizations can be expected to continue and probably increase their investment in outcomes research and similar activities, these efforts taken as a whole are unlikely to substitute for more than a portion of government-supported research and training in magnitude, coherence, scope, or concern for long-term consequences. Like other kinds of health-related research and training in the biomedical and clinical sciences, health services research and research training are, in considerable measure, public goods worthy of support by society as a whole.

References

AHCPR (Agency for Health Care Policy and Research). National Research Service Award Individual Postdoctoral Fellowships (Publication Number 94–0078). Rockville, Md.: Department of Health and Human Services, June, 1994.

AHCPR. National Research Service Award—Institutional Grants Policy and Guidelines (Publication Number 95–0013). Rockville, Md.: Department of Health and Human Services, December, 1994.

Anderson, O. *The Uneasy Equilibrium: Private and Public Financing of Health Services in the United States 1875–1965.* New Haven, Conn.: College and University Press, 1968.

Brook, R.H., and Lohr, K.N. Efficacy, Effectiveness, Variations, and Quality: Boundary–crossing Research. *Medical Care* 23:710–722, 1985.

Brook, R., Chassin, M., Park, R., et al. A Method for Detailed Assessment of the Appropriateness of Medical Technologies. *International Journal of Technology Assessment in Health Care* 2:53–63, 1986.

Brown, D. Small Agency Is a Target in Budgeting. *New York Times,* April 16, 1995, p. 17.

Browne, M.W. Supply Exceeds Demand for Ph.D.'s in Many Science Fields. *New York Times*, July 4, 1995, p. 16.

Capilouto, E., Capilouto, M.L., and Ohsfeldt, R. A Review of Methods Used to Project the Future Supply of Dental Personnel and the Future Demand and Need for Dental Services. *Journal of Dental Education* 59(1):237–257, 1995.

CCMC (Committee on the Costs of Medical Care). *Medical Care for the American People.* Chicago, Ill.: University of Chicago Press, 1932. (Reprinted by U.S. Department of Health, Education and Welfare, 1972.)

Chassin, M., Kosecoff, J., Park, R., et al. Does Inappropriate Use Explain Geographic Variations in the Use of Health Care Services? A Study of Three Procedures. *Journal of the American Medical Association* 258:2533–2537, 1987.

Codman, E.A. The Product of a Hospital. *Journal of Surgery, Gynecology, and Obstetrics* 18(4):491–496, 1914.

COSEPUP (Commission on Science, Engineering, and Public Policy) of the National Academy of Sciences, National Academy of Engineering, and Institute of Medicine. *Reshaping the Graduate Education of Scientists and Engineers.* Washington, D.C.: National Academy Press, 1995.

Densen, P.M., Shapiro, S. and Einhorn, M. Concerning High and Low Utilizers of Service in a Medical Care Plan, and the Persistence of Utilization Levels Over a Three-Year Period. *Milbank Memorial Fund Quarterly* 37:217-250, 1959.

Donabedian, A. Evaluating the Quality of Medical Care. *Milbank Memorial Fund Quarterly* 44:166–203, July (part 2) 1966.

Donabedian, A. *Explorations in Quality Assessment and Monitoring*; Vol. 1. *The Definition of Quality and Approaches to Its Assessment*; Vol. 2. *The Criteria and Standards of Monitoring*; Vol. 3. *The Methods and Findings of Quality Assessment and Monitoring: An Illustrated Analysis.* Ann Arbor, Mich.: Health Administration Press, 1980, 1982, 1985.

Ebert–Flattau, P., and Perkoff, G.T. The Health Services Research Labor Force in the United States. *Medical Care* 21:253–265, 1983.

Eddy, D. Oregon's Methods: Did Cost–effectiveness Analysis Fail? *Journal of the American Medical Association* 266:2135–2141, 1991.

Eddy, D., and Billings, J. The Quality of Medical Evidence: Implications for Quality of Care. *Health Affairs* 7:19–32, 1988.

Eisenberg, J. *Doctors' Decisions and the Cost of Medical Care: The Reasons for Doctors' Practice Patterns and the Ways to Change Them.* Ann Arbor, Mich.: Health Administration Press Perspectives, 1986.

Ellwood, P. Alternatives to Regulation: Improving the Market. In: *Controls on Health Care.* Papers of the Conference on Regulation in the Health Industry, January 7–9, 1974. Washington, D.C.: National Academy of Sciences, 1975, pp. 49–72.

Ellwood, P. Shattuck Lecture. Outcomes Management: A Technology of Patient Experience. *New England Journal of Medicine* 318:1549–1556, 1988.

Enthoven, A. Managed Competition: An Agenda for Action. *Health Affairs* 7(3):25–47, 1988.

Epstein, A.M. U.S. Teaching Hospitals in the Evolving Health Care System. *Journal of the American Medical Association* 273:1203–1207, 1995.

Feil, E.C., Welch, H.G., and Fisher, E.S. Why Estimates of Physician Supply and Requirements Disagree. *Journal of the American Medical Association* 269:2859–2863, 1993.

FHSR (Foundation for Health Services Research). *Directory of Training Programs in Health Services Research, 1991–1992.* Washington, D.C.: Foundation for Health Services Research, 1992.

Fifer, W.R. Quality Assurance in the Computer Era. In: N.O. Graham, *Quality Assurance in Hospitals: Strategies for Assessment and Implementation.* Rockville, Md.: Aspen Publishers, pp. 288–296, 1990.

Flook, E.E., and Sanazaro, P.J., eds. *Health Services Research and R&D in Perspective.* Ann Arbor, Mich.: Health Administration Press, 1973.

Gaus, C.R. Health Services Research: Now More than Ever. *Journal of the American Medical Association* 274:108, 1995.

Goldschmidt, P. G. Health Services Research and Development: The Veterans Administration Program. *Health Services Research* 20(6):789–824, 1986.

Gray, B.F. The Legislative Battle Over Health Services Research. *Health Affairs* 11:38–66, 1992.

Green, J., and Wintfeld, N. Report Cards on Cardiac Surgeons: Assessing New York State's Approach. *New England Journal of Medicine* 332:1229–1232, 1995.

Greenlick, M.R., Freeborn, D.K. and Pope, C.R. *Health Care Research in an HMO: Two Decades of Discovery.* Baltimore, Md.: The Johns Hopkins University Press, 1988.

Hadley, J., Steinberg, E.P., and Feder, J. Comparison of Uninsured and Privately Insured Hospital Patients. *Journal of the American Medical Association* 265:374–379, 1991.

Hannan, E.L., Kilburn, H., Racz, M., Shields, E., and Chassin, M. Improving the outcomes of coronary artery bypass surgery in New York State. *Journal of the American Medical Association.* 271(10): 761-6, 1994.

Harrington, C., and Newcomer, R.J. Social Health Maintenance Organizations' Service Use and Costs, 1985–89. *Health Care Financing Review* 12(3):37–52, 1991.

IOM (Institute of Medicine). *Health Services Research: Report of a Study.* Washington, D.C.: National Academy of Sciences, 1979.

IOM. *Personnel Needs and Training for Biomedical and Behavioral Research.* Washington, D.C.: National Academy Press, 1983.

IOM. *Personnel Needs and Training for Biomedical and Behavioral Research.* Washington, D.C.: National Academy Press, 1985.

IOM. *Controlling Costs and Changing Patient Care: The Role of Utilization Management.* Washington, D.C.: National Academy Press, 1989.

IOM. *Clinical Practice Guidelines: Directions for a New Program.* M.J. Field and K.N. Lohr, eds. Washington, D.C.: National Academy Press, 1990a.

IOM. *Medicare: A Strategy for Quality Assurance.* K. Lohr, ed. Washington, D.C.: National Academy Press, 1990b.

IOM. *Improving Information Services for Health Services Researchers. A Report to the National Library of Medicine.* J. Harris–Wehling and L.C. Morris, eds. Washington, D. C.: National Academy Press, 1991.

IOM *Guidelines for Clinical Practice: From Development to Use.* M.J. Field and K.N. Lohr, eds. Washington, D.C.: National Academy Press, 1992.

IOM. *Access to Health Care in America.* M. Millman, ed. Washington, D.C.: National Academy Press, 1993a.

IOM. *Employment and Health Benefits: A Connection at Risk.* M.J. Field and H.T. Shapiro, eds. Washington, D.C.: National Academy Press, 1993b.

IOM. *Balancing the Scales of Opportunity: Ensuring Racial and Ethnic Diversity in the Health Professions.* M.E. Lewin and B. Rice, eds. Washington, D.C.: National Academy Press, 1994a.

IOM. *Health Services Research: Opportunities for an Expanding Field of Inquiry. An Interim Statement.* S. Thaul, K.N. Lohr, and R.E. Tranquada, eds. Washington, D.C.: National Academy Press, 1994b.

IOM. *Dental Education at the Crossroads: Challenges and Change.* M.J. Field, ed. Washington, D.C.: National Academy Press, 1995.

Kane, R.L., and Blewett, L.A. Quality Assurance for a Program of Comprehensive Care for Older Persons. *Health Care Financing Review* 14:89–110, 1993.

Kindig, D.A. Counting Generalist Physicians. *Journal of the American Medical Association* 271:1505–1507, 1994.

Koen, M.E. Hospitals in Profile. *Inquiry* 2(2):43–58, 1965.

Langwell, K., Rossiter, L., Brown, R. et al. Early Experience of Health Maintenance Organizations Under Medicare Competition Demonstrations. *Health Care Financing Review* 8:37–55, 1987.

Lasker, R.D., Humphreys, B.L., and Braithwaite, W.R. Making a Powerful Connection: The Health of the Public and the National Information Infrastructure. Report of the U.S. Public Health Service Public Health Data Policy Coordinating Committee, Washington, D.C. July 6, 1995.

Lurie, M., Ward, N.B., Shapiro, M.F., et al. Termination from Medi–Cal: Does It Affect Health? *New England Journal of Medicine* 311:480–484, 1984.

Newhouse, J.P., and the Insurance Experiment Group. *Free for All?: Lessons from the RAND Health Insurance Experiment Group.* Cambridge, Mass.: Harvard University Press, 1993.

NRC (National Research Council). *Personnel Needs and Training for Biomedical and Behavioral Research.* Washington, D.C.: National Academy Press, 1975a.

NRC. Report of the Committee on a Feasibility Study of National Needs for Biomedical and Behavioral Research Personnel. Washington, D.C.: National Academy Pres, 1975b.

NRC. *Personnel Needs and Training for Biomedical and Behavioral Research.* Washington, D.C.: National Academy Press, 1976.

NRC. *Personnel Needs and Training for Biomedical and Behavioral Research.* Vol. 1. Washington, D.C.: National Academy Press, 1977.

NRC. *Personnel Needs and Training for Biomedical and Behavioral Research.* Washington, D.C.: National Academy Press, 1978.

NRC. *Personnel Needs and Training for Biomedical and Behavioral Research.* Washington, D.C.: National Academy Press, 1979.

NRC. *Personnel Needs and Training for Biomedical and Behavioral Research.* Washington, D.C.: National Academy Press, 1981.

NRC. *Personnel Needs and Training for Biomedical and Behavioral Research.* Washington, D.C.: National Academy Press, 1989.

NRC. *Meeting the Nation's Needs for Biomedical and Behavioral Scientists.* Washington, D.C.: National Academy Press, 1994.

NRC and IOM. *Toward a National Health Care Survey: A Data System for the 21st Century.* G.S. Wunderlich, ed. Washington, D.C.: National Academy Press, 1992.

Office of Technology Assessment. *Identifying Health Technologies That Work: Searching for Evidence.* Washington, D.C.: U.S. Government Printing Office, 1994.

PSAC (President's Science Advisory Committee), Office of Science and Technology, Executive Office of the President. *Improving Health Care Through Research and Development.* Washington, D.C.: Government Printing Office, March 1972.

Rorem, C.R. *A Quest for Certainty: Essays on Health Care Economics, 1930–1970.* Ann Arbor, Mich.: Health Administration Press, 1982.

Shortell, S.M., and Reinhardt, U.E., eds. *Improving Health Policy and Management: Nine Critical Research Issues for the 1990s.* Ann Arbor, Mich.: Health Administration Press, 1992.

Somers, H.M., and Somers, A.R. *Doctors, Patients, and Health Insurance.* Washington, D.C.: The Brookings Institution, 1961.

Starr, P. *The Social Transformation of American Medicine.* New York, N.Y.: Basic Books, 1982.

Steinwachs, D.M. Health Services Research: Its Scope and Significance. In: *Promoting Health Services Research in Academic Health Centers*, P. Forman, ed. Washington, D.C.: Association of Academic Health Centers, 1991.

University of California, Universitywide Health Sciences Committee. *Universitywide Health Sciences Applicant Pool Study and Outreach Program Inventory.* Vol. I: Executive Summary Findings. Oakland, Calif.: University of California, 1993.

USDHEW (U.S. Department of Health, Education, and Welfare). *Training Grants Program of the National Center for Health Services Research and Development: Policies and Guidelines for Applicants.* Bethesda, Md.: U.S. Department of Health, Education and Welfare, 1970.

Wennberg, J. Dealing with Medical Practice Variations: A Proposal for Action. *Health Affairs* 3:6–32, 1984.

Wennberg, J., and Gittelsohn, A. Variations in Medical Care Among Small Areas. *Scientific American* 246:120–134, 1982.

Young, L.A. From the Blue Shield Perspective. *Inquiry* 2:5–15, 1965.

A New Database on the
U.S. Health Services Research Work Force

Nancy Cross Dunham, Ph.D.[1]

BACKGROUND

Little current, definitive information exists about the size and characteristics of the U.S. health services research work force. This paper describes how a new database was created for the Institute of Medicine (IOM) Committee on Health Services Research: Training and Work Force Issues.

The last effort to gather systematic information on the health services research work force dates back to the late 1970s when the National Research Council (NRC) supported a survey of individuals who had received funding for health services research or training from the National Center for Health Services Research or the Alcohol, Drug Abuse and Mental Health Administration. That study identified 1,378 health services researchers.[2] A 1983 IOM report estimated that there were between 600 and 1,650 health services researchers in 1979.[3] The lower estimate was based on the membership of the Committee on Health Services Research of the Medical Care Section of the American Public Health Association, and the higher estimate was based on assumptions about growth in the group identified in 1977.

---

[1]Deputy Director, Wisconsin Network for Health Policy Research at the University of Wisconsin–Madison. This paper has been edited by IOM committee members and staff.

[2]Ebert-Flattau, P., and Perkoff, G.T. The Health Services Research Labor Force in the United States. *Medical Care* 21(3):253–265, 1983.

[3]Institute of Medicine. *Personnel Needs and Training for Biomedical and Behavioral Research,* Washington, D.C.: National Academy of Sciences, 1983.

More recently, the membership of the Association for Health Services Research (AHSR), now the major professional organization for the field, has been used as a proxy to estimate trends in the supply of health services researchers. For example, a 1993 report, commissioned by the NRC, noted that AHSR's membership grew from 450 in 1983 to about 2,000 members in 1992.[4]

DATA SOURCES AND PROCEDURES

The database created for the study started with the membership files of the AHSR ($n = 2,311$ in early 1995). The files included addresses and, sometimes, degree information. Not all health services researchers belong to AHSR, and some AHSR members support the organization but are not health services researchers.

A second major source of names was HSRProj ($n = 1,213$ at the end of 1994), a comprehensive database on health services research activities in the United States developed by the Foundation for Health Services Research and the Sheps Center for Health Services Research at the University of North Carolina at Chapel Hill. The database is now a part of the National Library of Medicine's system of on-line information resources. The database contains information on health services research projects funded by the federal government and by six major private foundations.[5] Limitations of the HSRProj database include the omission of researchers funded by smaller foundations and industry. In addition, only the principal investigators of the funded research projects are included on the database.

When the AHSR and HSRProj data were combined, duplicate names were dropped, as were listings for those who

- had addresses outside of the United States;
- indicated they were students on the AHSR membership application form; and
- did not self-identify as health services researchers on the AHSR membership application form.

---

[4]B.N. Davidson, "Personnel Needs and Training for Health Services Research," background paper prepared for the National Research Council's Committee on National Needs for Biomedical and Behavioral Research Personnel, Washington, D.C., 1993.

[5]The Pew Charitable Trusts, the Robert Wood Johnson Foundation, the John A. Hartford Foundation, the Henry J. Kaiser Family Foundation, the Commonwealth Fund, and the W.K. Kellogg Foundation.

The resulting data set included 2,200 names. To this database were then added (1) names for those registered for the 1992 and 1993 AHSR annual conferences (*n* = approximately 700 after elimination of duplicate names and those with foreign addresses); names listed in the brochures of about 50 university-based and private health research "centers" (*n* = approximately 250 after elimination of duplicate names); and a list of nurse researchers supplied by Sigma Theta Tau International, the nursing honor society (*n* = 789 before elimination of a small number of duplicate names, the exact number of which was not recorded).

The final source of names was a written survey of 496 organizational employers of health services researchers. The list of organizations was compiled from several sources including (1) AHSR's institutional membership list and individuals' organizational affiliations indicated on the AHSR and HSRProj databases, (2) the research "centers" mentioned above, (3) individuals' organizational affiliations indicated on the registration list for the 1994 meeting of the National Association of Health Data Organizations, and (4) lists of relevant federal and state government offices. Survey respondents were asked to supply the names, addresses, telephone numbers, and degrees of the people in their organizations whom they considered to be health services researchers, according to the IOM's definition (see Chapter 1). They were also asked about their current and planned recruiting efforts. Of the 496 organizations surveyed, 154 returned the survey form, for an overall response rate of 31 percent. Because the tight schedule precluded follow-up mailings to nonrespondents, this low response rate was not unexpected. The survey yielded a total of 1,731 names of health services researchers, about 970 of which were not already included in the database.

SUMMARY OF RESULTS

The final database included 4,920 names, more than double the membership of the AHSR. This list, however, still does not include all those engaged in the field, and it probably includes some individuals who would not self-identify or be identified by others as health services researchers.[6]

---

[6]If it were assumed that nonrespondents to the written survey employed health services researchers at the same rate as respondents, approximately 600 more researchers could be added to the database count.

Distribution of Researchers by Region and State

Table A.1 presents information on the distribution of the health services researchers in the *full* database by geographic region and state. Geographically, 27 percent of the researchers in the database are located in the South Atlantic region of the country, primarily because of the concentration of researchers in Maryland and the District of Columbia. The next highest concentrations of health services researchers are seen in the Pacific region (16 percent) and the East North Central region (16 percent). California, with 567 health services researchers, has the largest state contingent, followed by Maryland (423), the District of Columbia (321), Massachusetts (317), and Pennsylvania (305).

Graduate Education

The *full* database included information on graduate degrees for nearly two-thirds (3,203) of the researchers listed. Of this group, 52 percent had doctoral training (including 73 individuals with Sc.D. and 16 individuals with Ed.D. degrees). Another 28 percent had clinical degrees (of which approximately three-quarters were M.D.s).

Type of Employer

For analytic purposes, organizations responding to the *written* survey were grouped into the following categories: universities, proprietary and nonprofit health services research organizations and consulting firms, professional groups, health industry organizations (including managed care organizations, insurance companies, and pharmaceutical companies), and federal and state government agencies. Table A.2 presents information on the types of responding organizations and their reported employment of health services researchers. Universities (which comprised 30 percent of the responding organizations) reported the highest numbers of health services researchers, 41 percent of the total and 55 percent of the Ph.D.-level researchers reported. Again, given the low response rate, the percentages reported should be viewed with caution.

TABLE A.1 Number of Identified Health Services Researchers, by Region/State

Region/State	No.	% of Total	Region/State	No.	% of Total
New England	527	11	East North Central	761	16
Connecticut	80		Illinois	226	
Maine	45		Indiana	92	
Massachusetts	317		Michigan	134	
New Hampshire	34		Ohio	129	
Rhode Island	44				
Vermont	7		West North Central	335	7
			Iowa	48	
Middle Atlantic	694	14	Kansas	28	
New Jersey	118		Minnesota	136	
New York	271		Missouri	81	
Pennsylvania	305		Nebraska	26	
			North Dakota	11	
South Atlantic	1,336	27	South Dakota	5	
Delaware	5				
District of Columbia	321		Mountain	194	4
Florida	89		Arizona	40	
Georgia	86		Colorado	52	
Maryland	423		Idaho	3	
North Carolina	176		Montana	6	
South Carolina	37		Nevada	18	
Virginia	185		New Mexico	31	
West Virginia	14		Utah	38	
			Wyoming	6	
East South Central	109	2			
Alabama	57		Pacific	778	16
Kentucky	19		Alaska	1	
Mississippi	10		California	567	
Tennessee	23		Hawaii	13	
			Oregon	71	
West South Central	186	4	Washington	126	
Arkansas	27				
Louisiana	14				
Oklahoma	15				
Texas	130		TOTAL	4,920	101[a]

[a]Total does not sum to 100 because of rounding.

TABLE A.2 Reported Employment of Health Services Researchers (HSRs) by Organizational Type

Organizational Type	Responses to Questionnaire		HSRs Employed		Ph.D.-level HSRs Employed	
	No.	(%)	No.	(%)	No.	(%)
Universities	46	(30)	715	(41)	411	(55)
Research or consulting organizations	27	(18)	513	(30)	164	(22)
Federal/state government	45	(29)	266	(15)	74	(10)
Health industry[a]	14	(9)	130	(8)	60	(8)
Professional groups	22	(14)	107	(6)	40	(5)
TOTAL	154	(100)	1,731	(100)	749	(100)

[a]Includes managed care plans, insurers, pharmaceutical firms, and integrated systems.

Current and Future Hiring of Researchers

The *written* survey of employers of health services researchers also included two questions relating to the demand for health services researchers in 13 specific research areas as reported in Tables A.3 and A.4. Respondents were asked

• if, in the last few years, they have had difficulty in recruiting Ph.D.-level researchers for specific research areas; and
• if, in the next five years, they intended to recruit Ph.D.-level researchers in any of these areas and, if so, how many.

Table A.3 shows the number of responding organizations that reported having had difficulty in the last few years in recruiting qualified Ph.D.-level researchers in one or more of the research areas listed in the questionnaire. Overall, more than half of the responding organizations (83, or 54 percent) indicated that they have had problems recruiting Ph.D.-level health services researchers. Universities, which are heavy employers of Ph.D.s, were more likely to report such problems. Over two-thirds of universities (70 percent) reported having difficulties in at least one of these research areas.

TABLE A.3 Organizations Reporting Difficulties in Recruiting Ph.D.-Level Health Services Researchers in the Past Few Years, by Type

Organizational Type	Reported Difficulties No. (%)[a]
Universities	32 (70)
Research or consulting organizations	15 (56)
Federal/state government	20 (44)
Health industry[b]	6 (43)
Professional groups	10 (46)
TOTAL	83 (54)

[a]In at least one area of research.
[b]Includes managed care plans, insurers, pharmaceutical firms, and integrated systems.

Table A.4 shows the specific research areas in which these recruiting problems have been reported by responding organizations. The research areas have been rank-ordered in terms of the number of organizations reporting problems (not the number of positions for which difficulties were experienced). For five research areas, at least 15 percent of the responding organizations reported difficulty recruiting researchers in the last few years. The areas reportedas having presented the greatest problems are outcomes/health status measurement (23 percent), health economics (21 percent), biostatistics (20 percent), epidemiology (18 percent), and health policy analysis (16 percent).

Anticipated Future Demand

Table A.5 presents information on the numbers of responding organizations that reported that they expected to recruit Ph.D. researchers in the various research areas over the next five years. Sixty-one percent of responding organizations indicated that they anticipated recruiting health services researchers in at least one of these areas of research. Government agencies were the least likely to report such plans.

TABLE A.4 Rank Order of Research Areas in Which Recruiting Difficulties Were Reported

Research Areas	Reported Difficulties No. (%)[a]
Outcomes/health status measurement	35 (23)
Health economics	32 (21)
Biostatistics	31 (20)
Epidemiology	25 (18)
Health policy analysis	24 (16)
Medical informatics	17 (11)
Managed care research	14 (9)
Gerontology	13 (8)
Operations/decision analysis	10 (6)
Quality	9 (6)
Nursing research	8 (5)
Mental health research	6 (4)
Dental health research	4 (3)
Other[b]	17 (11)

[a]In at least one area of research. Many organizations reported difficulties in more than one area.
[b]Categories listed include actuarial science, bioethics, demography, health care management, health education, health finance, health services research (general), long-term care, pharmacy services research, modeling, and work force planning.

TABLE A.5 Number of Organizations Indicating Plans to Recruit Health Services Researchers in the Next Five Years

Organizational Type	Reported Plans No. (%)[a]
Universities	36 (78)
Research or consulting organizations	18 (67)
Federal/state government	16 (36)
Health industry[b]	13 (93)
Professional groups	11 (36)
TOTAL	94 (61)

[a]Reported plans to recruit people for at least one area of research.
[b]Includes managed care plans, insurers, pharmaceutical firms, and integrated systems.

Table A.6 indicates that the five research areas (outcomes/health status measurement, health economics, biostatistics, epidemiology, and health policy analysis) for which responding employers reported having had difficulty recruiting in the last few years are also the areas in which demand is anticipated to be strongest in the next five years. Based on the estimates of responding organizations, they will hire more than 660 health services researchers in the next five years.

TABLE A.6 Research Areas in Which Responding Organizations (n = 154) Expect to Recruit Health Services Researchers in the Next Five Years

Research Areas	Total Number of Researchers Expected to Be Recruited	
	No.	(%)
Outcomes/health status measurement	120	(18)
Health economics	96	(14)
Biostatistics	83	(13)
Epidemiology	71	(11)
Health policy analysis	62	(9)
Managed care research	49	(7)
Operations/decision analysis	39	(6)
Quality	38	(6)
Mental health research	26	(4)
Medical informatics	26	(4)
Nursing research	17	(3)
Gerontology	14	(2)
Dental health research	1	(<1)
Other	19	(3)
TOTAL	661	(100)

SUMMARY

To develop current estimates of the size of the health services research work force in the United States, a variety of sources were used to build a database. The process yielded a database containing information on a total of 4,920 individual health services researchers, a number considerably higher than past estimates. It is important to note, however, that the database is likely to include some individuals who are not health services researchers and to exclude some who are. Moreover, it lacks information (e.g., age) that would be useful in developing estimates of the future supply of researchers. Demand for health services researchers over the next five years is expected to continue, especially in universities and the health industry. Researchers with experience in outcomes/health status measurement, health economics, biostatistics, epidemiology, and health policy analysis will be in particular demand.

Survey of Health Services Research
Educational Programs[1]

OBJECTIVES AND METHOD

To obtain more information and perspectives on educational programs in health services research, the Institute of Medicine (IOM) Committee on Health Services Research Training and Work Force Issues decided at its first meeting in July 1995 to canvass these programs for additional information. The IOM then requested and received funding for this additional work from the Robert Wood Johnson Foundation. Funds from the Baxter Foundation also helped support this activity.

As a starting point, staff used the 121 health services research training programs in the United States and Canada that were listed in the 1991–1992 directory compiled by the Foundation for Health Services Research (FHSR). Although the listing is not all-inclusive, it was the most comprehensive one available to the committee. The list included information on 45 master's programs, 66 doctoral programs, and 26 fellowship programs for a total of 137. The sum of program categories exceeds 121 because some programs offer both a master's and a doctoral program.

In early December 1994, the programs listed in the FHSR directory were mailed (1) a copy of their entry in the 1991–1992 FHSR directory for updating and (2) a three-page, open-ended questionnaire developed by the committee. The questionnaire asked about program structure, students' academic and work backgrounds, curriculum, enrollment, financial aid, and post-training careers of graduates. Nonrespondents received follow-up phone calls to encourage them to

---

[1]This appendix was prepared by Jill Feasley of the project staff.

return the questionnaire. Sixty-three of the 137 programs returned questionnaires for an overall response rate of 46 percent.[2] (Responses were received from 18 master's, 30 doctoral, and 15 fellowship programs for response rates of 40, 45, and 58 percent respectively.) An additional 13 programs returned only their directory update.

FINDINGS

Program Structure

Reflecting the multidisciplinary nature of the health services research field, the structure and focus of health services research programs vary considerably. Some programs are devoted explicitly to health services research whereas others offer a health services research concentration within a distinct discipline such as nursing, pharmacy, or social work. Some programs are housed in their own academic departments, others draw from several departments in the university, and a few operate under the shared or primary auspices of institutions such as Veterans Affairs hospitals that are not universities. Table B.1 displays the areas and disciplines offering programs in health services research as categorized in the FHSR directory.

Many programs reported that they are considering changing or already have changed their programs from the traditional full-time, daytime, on-site format to include alternative offerings that better accommodate students who continue to work or are enrolled on a part-time basis. Classes are now being offered on evenings and weekends, by mail or other distance learning arrangements, and through summer institutes or other types of short and intensive courses. Some programs are specifically designed for business and government executives or midcareer professionals.

Academic and Work Backgrounds of Students

As might be expected, before entering the health services research educational programs, students had studied a variety of academic disciplines at both the undergraduate and graduate levels. Survey respondents most frequently cited student backgrounds in clinical areas (e.g., nursing, dentistry), with

---

[2]The timing of the survey may have contributed to the relatively low overall response rate; the survey was sent out just as most academic programs were finishing the first semester and starting the winter break. Beyond the follow-up phone calls, the study timetable did not allow for intensive follow up.

TABLE B.1 Doctoral and Postdoctoral Fellowship Programs in Health Service Research by Discipline and Degree Level, as categorized in the 1991–1992 Foundation for Health Services Research Directory

Discipline	Level[a]	Institution/Program
CLINICAL SCIENCE		
General	Doctoral	University of California, Berkeley, San Francisco/Health Services Research Training Program
	Fellowship	University of California, Berkeley, San Francisco/Health Services Research Training Program
Medicine	Doctoral	Dartmouth University/Ph.D. in the Evaluative Clinical Sciences
	Fellowship	Stanford University/Veterans Affairs (VA) Medical Center Research Fellowship in Ambulatory Care
Internal medicine	Doctoral	Seattle VA/VA Ambulatory Care Fellowship
Preventive	Fellowship	Mt. Sinai School of Medicine/Fellowship in General Preventive Medicine
	Fellowship	University of Washington/Postdoctoral Fellowship in the Prevention of Chronic Diseases
Geriatrics	Fellowship	Brown University/Health Services Research Fellowship in Geriatrics and Gerontology
Epidemiology	Doctoral	Brown University/Ph.D. in Epidemiology and Gerontology
Family medicine	Fellowship	University of Medicine and Dentistry of New Jersey, Robert Wood Johnson Medical School/Health Services Research and Policy Fellowship
Pediatrics	Fellowship	University of Rochester/General Pediatrics Research Fellowship
Nursing	Doctoral	Boston College/Ph.D. in Nursing
	Doctoral	Case Western Reserve University/Ph.D. in Nursing
	Doctoral	Catholic University of America/Ph.D. in Nursing
	Doctoral	George Mason University/Ph.D. in Nursing Administration
	Doctoral	Indiana University/Ph.D. in Nursing Administration
	Doctoral	University of Alabama in Birmingham/Ph.D. in Nursing
	Doctoral	University of Colorado School of Nursing/Ph.D. in Nursing
	Doctoral	University of Iowa/Ph.D. in Nursing Administration
	Doctoral	University of Kansas/Ph.D. in Nursing

continued

TABLE B.1 Continued

Discipline	Level	Institution/Program
Nursing (continued)	Doctoral	University of Maryland School of Nursing/Ph.D. in Nursing
	Doctoral	University of Pennsylvania/Ph.D. in Nursing
	Doctoral	University of Rochester/Ph.D. in Nursing
	Fellowship	Case Western Reserve University/Doctoral Program in Nursing
Pharmacy	Doctoral	University of North Carolina at Chapel Hill/Ph.D. in Pharmacy Administration
	Doctoral	University of Maryland School of Pharmacy/Ph.D. in Pharmacy Administration
	Doctoral	University of Texas at Austin/Ph.D. in Pharmacy Administration
Social work	Doctoral	University of Denver/Ph.D. in Social Work
	Doctoral	University of Maryland School of Social Work/Ph.D. in Social Work
	Doctoral	Washington University/Ph.D. in Social Work
	Fellowship	University of Tennessee/Ph.D. Program in Social Work
PUBLIC HEALTH	Doctoral	Columbia University/Ph.D. in Public Health
	Doctoral	Columbia University/Ph.D. in Sociomedical Science
	Doctoral	University of Iowa/Ph.D. in Health Management and Policy: Dental Public Health
SOCIAL SCIENCES	Doctoral	Brandeis University/Ph.D. in Health Policy
	Doctoral	Claremont Graduate School/Ph.D. in Psychology
	Doctoral	Indiana University/Ph.D. in Economics
	Doctoral	Johns Hopkins University/Health Services Research Training
	Doctoral	Johns Hopkins University/Ph.D. in Economics and Mental Health
	Doctoral	New York University/Ph.D. in Public Administration
	Doctoral	Northwestern University/Health Services Research Doctoral Concentration Program
	Doctoral	Pennsylvania State University/Ph.D. in Health Policy and Administration

SOCIAL SCIENCES (continued)

	Doctoral	RAND/University of California, Los Angeles (UCLA) Center for Health Policy Study/Policy Career Development Program
	Doctoral	Stanford University/Ph.D. in Medical Information Sciences
	Doctoral	State University of New York at Binghamton/Ph.D. in Political Science with Emphasis on Policy Analysis
	Doctoral	St. Louis University/Ph.D. in Health Services Research
	Doctoral	University of California, Berkeley/Ph.D. Program in Social Welfare
	Doctoral	University of California, Berkeley/Ph.D. in Health Services and Policy Analysis
	Doctoral	University of California, Berkeley/Economics of Aging and Health Services Research Training Program
	Doctoral	University of California, Berkeley–San Francisco/Health Services Research Training Program
	Doctoral	University of California, Los Angeles/Ph.D. in Health Services
	Doctoral	University of California, Los Angeles/Ph.D. in Social Welfare
	Doctoral	University of California, San Francisco/Ph.D. in Sociology
	Doctoral	University of Illinois at Urbana-Champaign/Medical Scholars Program
	Doctoral	University of Maryland Graduate School/Ph.D. in Policy Sciences
	Doctoral	University of Michigan/Ph.D. in Health Services Organization and Policy
	Doctoral	University of Minnesota/Ph.D. in Health Services Research, Policy and Administration
	Doctoral	University of North Carolina at Chapel Hill/Predoctoral Training Program in Health Services Research and Policy Analysis
	Doctoral	University of Pennsylvania/Ph.D. in Health Care Systems
	Doctoral	University of Texas at Austin/Ph.D. in Pharmacy Administration
	Doctoral	University of Wisconsin–Madison/Ph.D. in Health Services Research
	Doctoral	University of Wisconsin–Madison/Ph.D. in Economics of Health/Mental Health
	Doctoral	Vanderbilt University/Ph.D. Program in Economics

continued

TABLE B.1 Continued

Discipline	Level	Institution/Program
SOCIAL SCIENCES (continued)	Doctoral	Virginia Commonwealth University/Ph.D. in Health Services Organization and Research
	Doctoral	Yale University/Ph.D. in Health Policy, Resources and Administration
	Fellowship	Harvard University/Postdoctoral Fellowships in Health Services Research
	Fellowship	Harvard University/Ph.D. in Health Policy
	Fellowship	Johns Hopkins University/Training in Health Services Research
	Fellowship	University of Maryland Center for Health Services Research/Public Academic Liaison Postdoctoral Fellowship in Mental Health Services Research
	Fellowship	Seattle VA Medical Center/Robert Wood Johnson Clinical Scholars Program
	Fellowship	University of California, Berkeley/Economics of Aging and Health Services Research Training Program
	Fellowship	University of California, Berkeley, San Francisco/Health Services Research Training Program
	Fellowship	University of California–San Francisco/Pew Health Policy Program
	Fellowship	University of California–San Francisco/Fellowship in Reproductive Health Policy
	Fellowship	University of California–Berkeley–San Francisco/ Health Services Research Training Program
	Fellowship	University of Medicine and Dentistry of New Jersey/Health Services Research and Policy Fellowship
	Fellowship	University of North Carolina–Chapel Hill/Postdoctoral Training Program in Health Services Research and Policy Analysis
	Fellowship	Durham VA Medical Center/Health Service Research and Development Fellowship
	Fellowship	Hines VA Hospital/Doctoral Training Program in Health Services Research
	Fellowship	Houston VA Medical Center/Quality of Care and Utilization Studies Doctoral Training

MANAGEMENT	Doctoral	George Washington University/Ph.D. in Health Services Management
	Doctoral	Georgia State University/Ph.D. in Risk Management and Insurance
	Doctoral	Northwestern University/Health Services Research Doctoral Concentration Program
	Doctoral	Pennsylvania State University/Doctoral Program in Health Policy and Administration
	Doctoral	Purdue University/Pharmacy Administration
	Doctoral	Stanford University/Medical Information Sciences Program
	Doctoral	Union College/Administrative and Engineering Systems Doctoral Program
	Doctoral	University of Alabama–Birmingham/Ph.D. in Administration–Health Services
	Doctoral	University of Illinois at Urbana–Champaign/Medical Scholars Program
	Doctoral	University of Iowa/Doctoral Studies in Health Management and Policy
	Doctoral	University of North Carolina–Chapel Hill/Ph.D. in Health Policy and Administration
	Doctoral	University of Oklahoma/Ph.D. in Health Administration and Policy
	Doctoral	University of Pennsylvania/Ph.D. in Nursing
	Doctoral	University of Pennsylvania/Health Care Systems Ph.D. Program
	Doctoral	University of South Carolina/Ph.D. in Pharmacy Administration
	Doctoral	University of Texas–Austin/Ph.D. in Nursing
	Doctoral	University of Wisconsin–Madison/Ph.D. in Health Systems Engineering
	Fellowship	Stanford University/Medical Information Sciences Program

[a]The categorization for master's programs is not presented in this table, although it was provided in the FHSR directory.

SOURCE: Foundation for Health Services Research. *Directory of Training Programs in Health Services Research, 1991–1992*. Washington, D.C.: Foundation for Health Services Research, 1992.

business, administration, and social sciences the next most frequently mentioned (Table B.2).

Survey respondents indicated that both master's and doctoral students have often had some type of work experience in health care (Table B.3). Respondents for doctoral programs also cited student work experiences in administration or research. Relatively few students were described as "preservice" (i.e., entering a program without any work experience), and most of these were master's-level students.

Curriculum

Respondents were asked to identify the core courses for a standard health services research curriculum. The only course cited by a majority of survey respondents for all program levels (master's, doctoral, and fellowship) was research methods, although majorities or near majorities also cited statistics or biostatistics (Table B.4). Health economics was another quantitatively oriented course cited by at least one-third of respondents in each program area. Health care organization was mentioned by the less than one-third of respondents in each of the program areas, although larger proportions mentioned health policy, which may have considerable overlap in course content.

In addition to the standard coursework, respondents noted the need for students to be involved in "real world" research under the supervision of a mentor. Ideally, the student should be involved with all phases of the research—from initial development to final dissemination. If students plan a career in academia, they should also write articles for scholarly journals and present academic papers at professional conferences. Students who will go on to conduct research should be involved with proposal writing and fundraising.

Enrollment

Building on information from the 1991–1992 FHSR directory and the responses to the canvass of educational programs, the committee attempted to develop a rough estimate of the health services research pipeline, that is, those who are students in health services research educational programs. For the 76 respondents who submitted an update of the FHSR directory information, the committee used their report of the number of students enrolled in each class. For the 45 respondents who did not return the update, the committee used the enrollment information reported in the 1991–1992 FHSR directory. For the former group, the committee compared their updated and earlier figures and found little change in enrollments for most programs, but the pattern for nonrespondents might be different.

TABLE B.2 Number and Percentage of Survey Respondents Indicating Typical Academic Backgrounds of Their Health Services Research Students

Academic Discipline	Master's Programs No. (%)	Doctoral Programs No. (%)	Fellowship Programs No. (%)
Clinical sciences	14 (82)	15 (58)	9 (64)
Business/administration	4 (24)	11 (42)	1 (7)
Social sciences	3 (18)	4 (15)	3 (21)
Public health	1 (6)	4 (15)	2 (14)
Other	4 (24)	6 (23)	7 (50)

NOTE: Number of programs responding to this question were as follows: master's, 17; doctoral, 26; and fellowship, 14. The percentages given are based on the number of programs responding to this question, not on the total number of programs responding to the survey. Respondents could list more than one response.

The combined figures on enrollment in each class from the two data sources show approximately 1,015 master's students, 511 doctoral students, and 197 postdoctoral fellows. As an estimate of the health services research pipeline, this number must be interpreted cautiously. On the one hand, for the master's level and other programs that offer concentrations in areas in addition to health services research, the numbers may include students who have concentrations other than health services research. On the other hand, the numbers refer to enrollments in each class, not to total enrollments.[3]

---

[3]To obtain an estimate of total enrollment, the committee considered multiplying the enrollment figure for each program by the reported years to complete a degree (two years for most master's-level programs and four to five years for doctoral programs). If the latter average were applied to the figure for doctoral enrollment reported in the text (511), it would yield an estimated 2,555 doctoral students in the pipeline. Based on committee members' involvement in the field, this number seemed implausibly high, presumably because it would not account for attrition. By way of contrast, for medical and dental school, enrollments are reported for the first through fourth years of school as well as for those graduating in a year (IOM, 1995).

TABLE B.3 Number and Percentage of Survey Respondents Indicating Typical Work Backgrounds of Their Health Services Research Students

Work Experience	Master's Programs No. (%)	Doctoral Programs No. (%)	Fellowship Programs No. (%)
Health care	16 (94)	20 (80)	7 (50)
Research	1 (6)	6 (24)	3 (21)
Preservice[a]	5 (29)	1 (4)	2 (14)
Administration	0 (0)	7 (28)	0 (0)
Academia	0 (0)	0 (0)	4 (29)
Other	2 (12)	6 (24)	3 (21)

NOTE: Number of programs responding to this question were as follows: master's, 17; doctoral, 25; and fellowship, 14. The percentages given are based on the number of programs responding to this question, not on the total number of programs responding to the survey. Respondents could list more than one response.

[a]The student had no prior work experience before entering the program.

Financial Aid

All of the doctoral and fellowship training programs reported offering some type of financial aid to some or all of their students, as do almost all of the master's-level programs. The amount of aid, however, varies considerably from program to program. For example, some doctoral programs reported offering a $15,000 stipend and free tuition to all students. Others can only waive the tuition for a few students in each class. In general, the fellowship programs are able to provide a higher stipend (the amounts reported ranged from $17,000 to $40,000), but usually the stipend is considerably less than the participant could be earning in his or her chosen field. The amount of support provided to master's-level students ranges from none to $14,000 plus a tuition waiver.

Survey respondents most frequently cited their university as a source of funding for student stipends (Table B.5) The federal government was the next most-often-cited source with financing coming either through explicit education awards such as the National Research Service Award or through research grants to the training institution that allow students to be hired for research projects. Foundations, state government, and private industry also provide funding to trainees. In particular, the Robert Wood Johnson Foundation and Pew Charitable Trusts have supported health services research and related educational programs.

TABLE B.4 Number and Percentage of Survey Respondents Indicating Core Courses for a Standard Health Service Research Curriculum

Course	Master's Programs No. (%)		Doctoral Programs No. (%)		Fellowship Programs No. (%)	
Research methods	11	(73)	22	(100)	6	(55)
Statistics/ Biostatistics	7	(47)	11	(50)	7	(64)
Health economics	6	(40)	12	(55)	4	(36)
Health policy	4	(27)	8	(36)	6	(55)
Epidemiology	5	(33)	4	(18)	7	(64)
Health care organization	3	(20)	7	(32)	3	(27)
Administration/ Management	3	(20)	3	(14)	1	(9)
Ethics	1	(7)	3	(14)	1	(9)
Other	6	(40)	5	(23)	4	(36)

NOTE: Number of programs responding to this question were as follows: master's, 15; doctoral, 22; and fellowship, 11. The percentages are based on the number of programs responding to this question, not on the total number of programs responding to the survey. Respondents could list more than one response.

Post-Training Careers

According to survey respondents, graduates of health services research training programs will go on to work in three general capacities: as a faculty member of an academic institution; as a researcher for an independent research organization; or as a policy analyst or researcher with a government agency. Others work in clinical or administrative settings, although the responses do not make clear the extent to which they are actually involved in research rather than patient care or management (Table B.6). Survey respondents indicated that graduates generally continue to hold the same types of jobs five years after completing their academic training.

TABLE B.5 Number and Percentage of Survey Respondents Indicating Source of Funding for Health Service Research Students' Stipends

Source of Funding	Master's Programs No. (%)		Doctoral Programs No. (%)		Fellowship Programs No. (%)	
University	12	(86)	21	(81)	4	(27)
Federal government	6	(43)	11	(42)	12	(80)
Grants, otherwise unspecified	1	(7)	5	(19)	0	(0)
State government	2	(14)	3	(12)	2	(13)
Foundation	3	(21)	2	(8)	4	(27)
Industry	3	(21)	2	(8)	2	(13)
Other	0	(0)	1	(4)	0	(0)

NOTE: Number of programs responding to this question were as follows: master's, 14; doctoral, 26; and fellowship, 15. The percentages given are based on the number of programs responding to this question, not on the total number of programs responding to the survey. Respondents could list more than one response.

TABLE B.6 Number and Percentage of Survey Respondents Indicating Post-Training Employment Settings of Graduates in Health Services Research

Employment Setting	Master's Programs No. (%)		Doctoral Programs No. (%)		Fellowship Programs No. (%)	
Academic institution	6	(38)	23	(92)	10	(77)
Research organization	9	(56)	17	(68)	7	(54)
Government agency	6	(38)	8	(32)	6	(46)
Clinical setting	3	(19)	1	(4)	2	(15)
Administrative setting	1	(6)	4	(16)	0	(0)
Not applicable/too new to know	4	(25)	0	(0)	1	(8)

NOTE: Number of programs responding to this question were as follows: master's, 16; doctoral, 25; and fellowship, 13. The percentages given are based on the number of programs responding to this question, not on the total number of programs responding to the survey. Respondents could list more than one response.

Multistate Life Table
Methodology and Projections[1]

Multistate period life tables were used in this report to develop projections of numbers of new Ph.D.s that would be needed in the future to sustain certain growth rates of the labor force. This Appendix describes briefly the method used to generate these results.[1]

Life table techniques are sometimes the only way to obtain estimates of certain statistics describing mobility and career characteristics of a population, especially those related to rates of occurrence of events, duration of time spent in an activity, and rates of attrition or exit from a population (due to death, retirement, job changing, etc.) even when we have not observed the full lifetimes of the scientists with our data (which is often the case with most data sets).[2] Moreover, life table methods provide a useful way of organizing various age-specific rates (rates of entering the labor force, changing jobs, moving abroad, retiring, and dying) into a logical framework, which can then be used to make projections of various characteristics of a population, such as its age distribution.

Multistate life tables, an extension of basic life tables, allow greater complexity to enter the analysis: people can enter as well as exit a population and can move back and forth across a variety of states within a population. Life

---

[1]This originally appeared as Appendix G in the National Research Council report *Meeting the Nation's Needs for Biomedical and Behavioral Scientists.* Washington, D.C.: National Academy Press, 1994.

tables may be classified as period versus cohort life tables. The Panel on Estimation Procedures decided that it was more practical, for the purposes of making projections, to use the former.

Construction of period life tables involves taking age-specific transition rates (job changing, unemployment, retirement, and death rates) prevailing during a particular period (e.g., 1989–1991) and applying them to a hypothetical (synthetic) cohort of people (actually a "synthetic" cohort of new Ph.D.s). Probabilities are then calculated of entrance or exit from a state (probability of entering a postdoctoral position, for example) and length of time spent in various states, as implied by the life table. Statistics of interest were developed for three time periods (1985–1991, 1979–1985, 1973–1979). Period life table results are conventionally referred to as "expected" quantities (i.e., "expected fraction of people who . . .," "expected length of time . . .") because of the nature of the methodology: constructing a single hypothetical Ph.D. cohort that experiences the current transition rates taken from a variety of Ph.D. cohorts.

The data for the life table analysis come from the longitudinal Survey of Doctorate Recipients (SDR), a sample survey that follows a group of Ph.D.s over time, interviewing basically the same people every 2 years. A general description follows (for details, see NRC, 1991 SDR Methodological Report, forthcoming). In 1973 an initial sample of science or engineering Ph.D.s living in the United States was drawn, and those sample members have been followed through time. New Ph.D.s enter the SDR in 1975 and each subsequent SDR year (1977, 1979, . . . 1991) and are followed over time as well. Individuals are followed until they reach a certain cutoff point that depends on the survey year at which they entered [typically 42 years after the Ph.D., although in recent SDR waves, they are followed until they reach age 70 or until they drop out for other reasons (nonresponse or death)].

The form of the data on which the life tables are based consists mostly of large sets of transition tables constructed from the SDR by National Research Council (NRC) staff (but death rates are obtained from TIAA-CREF data from the late 1980s, taken from Bowen and Sosa, 1991). For every pair of biennial survey-interview years ("waves") in the SDR (1973–1975 as the first pair, 1989–1991 as the last pair), the number of people moving between various states within those 2 years were obtained. These states were: postdoctorate, R&D employment[3] within one's broad Ph.D. field (biomed, behavioral, other), non-R&D employment within broad Ph.D. field, employment outside of broad Ph.D. field, out of labor force or unemployed (combined), leaving the country, retirement, and death. All of the biennial transition proportions were obtained by 2-year age group by broad Ph.D. field, and by sex. The survey observations (i.e., people) in one set of biennial transitions are often the same people in subsequent sets (though older).[4]

Another data ingredient for the life tables is the distribution of states (same as above) of "new entrants to the SDR" for SDR waves 1975–1991, again by age, sex, and Ph.D. field. These are used as estimates of numbers of new Ph.D.s in each survey year.

These transition data sets constructed by NRC staff were transformed into proportions to be used as input into a Multistate Life Table program (Tiemeyer and Ulmer, 1991). Initial work involved explorations of data quality, sample sizes, and the stability of rates over time. To have large enough sample sizes for (what we would hope to be) reliable estimates of sex differences in career patterns as well as estimates of how the career patterns have changed over time, it was necessary to aggregate the data into three broad time periods (as opposed to looking at a larger number of time periods): 1985–1991, 1979–1985, 1973–1979.

Projection Models

Life table construction begins by calculating a matrix containing the proportion of individuals exiting an origin state for each possible destination state between ages x and x+2 (in our case). This matrix is called $\mathbf{M_x}$.

Our projection models hold the population of those employed "in field" to some constant growth rate. The following algorithm is used:

1. Survive the current specified Ph.D. population forward 2 years.
2. Calculate the number of individuals employed "in field."
3. Calculate the differences between the target "in field" population and the number "in field" in the survived current population. This yields the number of new entrants needed to increase the "in field" population to its target size.
4. Divide the result of (3) by the proportion of new entrants who enter an "in field" employment state on receiving their Ph.D.
5. Use the result of (4) as the number of new entrants who would have had to enter the population between year y and y+2 to attain the target "in field" population. Add these individuals into the life table, distributed approximately by age and destination state.

Let $N_{x,y}$ represent the number of individuals in the specified Ph.D. population in each employment state at age X for a given year Y. $N_{x,y}$ is a k by k matrix, where k equals the number of states in the model. The columns indicate origin states (in the base year) and the rows destination states. So $N_{x,1995}[4,1]$ would equal the number of people who were in the 4th state (out of field employment) in 1995 who were in the 1st state (in field post-doc) in 1991.

For the base year, the off-diagonal elements of $N_{x,1991}$ are all 0 and the on-diagonal elements are equal the number of individuals age X in 1991 in the specified Ph.D. population in each employment state.

Let $N^-_{x,y}$ represent the number of individuals in each state (by origin state in 1991) in year y, BEFORE new entrants between year y and y–2 are added into the life table. Then $N^-_{x,y}$ is given by:

$$N^-_{x,y} = N_{x,y-2} \cdot \left(I + \frac{M_x}{2}\right)^{-1} \cdot \left(I - \frac{M_x}{2}\right)$$

Let F_{1991} represent the total number of individuals in the specified Ph.D. population employed "in field" in year 1991. Then F_{1991} is given by:

$$F_{1991} = \sum_{x=25}^{71} \sum_{o=1}^{3} \sum_{d=1}^{8} N_{x,1991}[d,o]$$

where x represents age, o represents origin of state, d represents destination state, $N_{x,1991}[o,d]$ represents the dth row and the oth column of $N_{x,1991}$, and where states 1 through 3 represent the employed "in field" states.

Let F^-_y represent the total number of individuals in the specified Ph.D. population employed "in field" in year Y who were in the specified Ph.D. population (although not necessarily employed "in field") in year Y–2. Then F^-_y is given by:

$$F^-_y = \sum_{x=25}^{71} \sum_{o=1}^{3} \sum_{d=1}^{8} N^-_{x,y}[d,o]$$

Let G represent the assumed 2-year growth rate for F_y. Then the target employed "in field" population size for any given year is:

Target "In Field" Population Size (y) =

$$F_{1991} \cdot (1+G)^{y \cdot 1991}$$

Let D_x represent the proportionate distribution by age and state of new entrants to the specified Ph.D. population over the two year period between Y and Y+2. D_x is a 1 by k vector with each column representing the proportion of all new entrants who are age X who enter that state on receiving their Ph.D. Summing D_x across all ages and states should equal one.

Finally, let R represent the proportion of all new entrants who enter an "in field" state on receiving their Ph.D. Then R is given by:

$$R = \sum_{x=25}^{71} \sum_{d=1}^{3} D_x[d]$$

Given $N_{x,1991}$, M_x, D_x, and G, then $N_{x,y}$ can be calculated for any y greater than 1991 (in increments of 2 years) by iterating through the formula:

$$N_{x,y|1991} =$$

$$N_x^- + \frac{((F_{1991} \cdot (1+G)^{y-1991}) - F_y^-)}{R} \cdot ((S \cdot D_x) x I)$$

which expands to:

$$N_{x,y|y>1991} = N_{x,y-2} \cdot \left(I + \frac{M_x}{2}\right)^{-1} \cdot \left(I - \frac{M_x}{2}\right) +$$

$$\frac{\left(F_{1991} \cdot (1+G)^{y-1991}\right) - \sum_{x=25}^{71} \sum_{o=1}^{3} \sum_{d=1}^{8} \left(N_{x,y-2} \cdot \left(I + \frac{M_x}{2}\right)^{-1} \cdot \left(I - \frac{M_x}{2}\right)\right)[d,o]}{R}$$

$$\cdot ((S \cdot D_x) x I)$$

where I is a k by k identity matrix, S is a k by 1 vector of ones, and the symbol x designates an element-wise matrix multiplication operation. (The operation ((S · D) x I) merely takes the D_x vector and turns it into a matrix with the elements of D_x on the main diagonal and zeros on the off diagonals).

The total number of new entrants is given by the component:

$$\frac{\left(F_{1991}\cdot(1+G)^{y-1991}\right)-\sum_{x=25}^{71}\sum_{o=1}^{3}\sum_{d=1}^{8}\left(N_{x,y-2}\cdot\left(I+\frac{M_x}{2}\right)^{-1}\cdot\left(I-\frac{M_x}{2}\right)\right)[d,o]}{R}$$

$$\cdot\left((S\cdot D_x)\times I\right)$$

Projections were made separately for each of 4 populations:

- biomedical Ph.D.s in biomedical employment fields,
- non–biomedical Ph.D.s in biomedical employment fields,
- behavioral Ph.D.s in behavioral employment fields, and
- non–behavioral Ph.D.s in behavioral employment fields.

To illustrate the use of life table analysis in generating projections of workforce variables, the Panel, as an exploratory exercise, chose to generate estimates of job openings. Given the uncertainty associated with efforts to project demand, the Panel examined three growth rates scenarios based on the average annual growth in the biomedical and behavioral science workforces between 1981 and 1991: zero growth; one-half the 1981–1991 average annual growth; and the average annual growth.[5] Estimates of "net separations"[6] were generated using the life tables. Estimates of needed job openings for the alternative growth scenarios were derived by adding to these separations the number of additional job openings that would need to be created to attain the particular target rate of growth.

In generating the estimates of job openings, the following assumptions were made:

1. There is never a negative number of new entrants. If there is a surplus in the employed "in field" population at a given year, no new entrants are added to the life table for that year.

2. The ratio of behavioral Ph.D.s to non–behavioral Ph.D.s employed in behavioral fields remains constant. That is, both Ph.D. populations increase or decrease at the same rate. The same assumption is made for the models of biomedical and non–biomedical Ph.D.s in biomedical employment.

3. The age/destination state proportionate distribution, D_x, is taken from the age/destination distribution observed among new entrants between 1985 and 1991.

4. The age/origin state distribution for the current population, $N_{x,1991}$, is calculated by taking the age-specific origin state distribution among the current Ph.D. population between 1985 and 1991 and applying it to the age distribution of the 1991 current population.

5. The age-specific 2-year transition proportions, M_x, used to survive the current age–distribution is taken from the observed transition proportions between 1985 and 1991.

NOTES

1. Methodological detail is available on request from NRC/OSEP Studies and Surveys Unit (Memorandum by Peter Tiemeyer, September 30, 1993). A general discussion of multistate life tables can be found in Keyfitz (1985).

2. In our particular project, however, we began with transition rates as the basic input data, and derived other life table statistics from those rates.

3. We define R&D employment to be basic or applied research, management of R&D, or development and design of systems and products; it is based on the individual's self-report of primary or secondary work activity.

4. With respect to the treatment of missing data: in general, to enter into the calculation of a biennial transition table, an individual case was required to have valid survey data on age and Ph.D. field and valid data for both of the survey years (for that transition table) on employment field (biomedical, behavioral, etc.) and employment status (postdoctorate, employed, retired, etc.). We developed decision rules for the treatment of all of these variables to handle various conditions (available on request). For example, work activity (i.e., R&D vs. non-R&D) could be missing if the person's employment field was other than biomedical or behavioral (because one of the "states" of the model is "employed outside of Ph.D. field" and those who are out of labor force, retired, or out of the country could be missing employment field and "work activity."

5. The 1981–1991 average annual growth rates were: 4.25 percent per year for the biomedical sciences workforce and 3.5 percent per year for the behavioral sciences workforce.

6. Net separations are defined in this analysis as losses arising from death, retirement or outmobility to another state minus gains from inmobility of experienced scientists from other states of employment. Alternative definitions will be explored in subsequent work by the Panel on Estimation Procedures.

REFERENCES

Bowen, W.G., and J.A. Sosa. 1989. *Prospects for Faculty in the Arts and Sciences.* Princeton, NJ: Princeton University Press.

Keyfitz, N. 1985. *Applied Mathematical Demography.* 2nd Ed. New York: Springer-Verlag.

National Research Council. Forthcoming. *1991 SDR Methodological Report.* Washington, D.C.: National Academy Press.

Tiemeyer, P., and G. Ulmer. 1991. *MSLT: A Program for the Computation of Multistate Life Tables.* Center for Demography Working Paper 91-34, University of Wisconsin.

Committee Biographies

ROBERT E. TRANQUADA, M.D., is Norman Topping/National Medical Enterprises Professor of Medicine and Public Policy at the University of Southern California (USC). Dr. Tranquada came to USC after receiving his M.D. degree from Stanford (1955) and completing his internship and residency in internal medicine at the University of California in 1959. He has held a number of progressively more responsible positions at USC and founded the Department of Community Medicine and Public Health in 1966. Dr. Tranquada also established and directed the Watts Health Center from 1965 to 1969. He was the dean of the School of Medicine from 1986 to 1991. Dr. Tranquada is a member of the Institute of Medicine and a fellow of the American Association for the Advancement of Science. He received the Association Distinguished Alumni Award from Stanford Medical Alumni in 1990. Dr. Tranquada is the author of over 50 scientific and educational papers and book chapters.

PAULA K. DIEHR, Ph.D., is Professor of Biostatistics and Health Services at the University of Washington. She spent 1975 to 1976 as a researcher at the Agency for Health Care Policy and Research (AHCPR). She has been a member of the Health Care Technology study section for AHCPR and of the Mental Health Services study section for the National Institute of Mental Health and is currently an advisor to the Office of Technology Assessment study on health insurance and access. She served on the editorial board of *Medical Care* and is currently on the editorial board of *Health Services Research*. She has presented several Association for Health Service Research (AHSR) workshops on analysis of utilization data and on small-area variation analysis. Dr. Diehr has worked almost exclusively in health services research, beginning with the Seattle Prepaid

Health Care Project in the early 1970s. Since then she has been involved in research about the use of health services, with a special emphasis on mental health services; different insurance and provider plans; health status; diagnostic rules for headache, cough and ankle trauma; health services for older adults; people without health insurance; survey methods; and evaluation of community-based health promotion programs. Her recent article on small-area variation analysis received the 1991 AHSR award for Article of the Year.

DEBORAH A. FREUND, M.P.H., Ph.D., is Vice-Chancellor for Academic Affairs and Dean of the Faculties at Indiana University, Bloomington (IU). She has served as special advisor to the president of the IU system. She is Professor of Public Affairs in Health Economics in the School of Public and Environmental Affairs and holds appointments in the Departments of Economics and Internal Medicine. In addition she directs the Otis Bowen Research Center at IU.

She received her M.A., M.P.H., and Ph.D. degrees in public health and economics at the University of Michigan and then embarked on a career in the administrative, policy, and research sectors. After managing the ambulatory care and surgery departments of a major teaching hospital and holding positions in federal and state government, she moved to the University of North Carolina at Chapel Hill where she spent nine years as a faculty member in its School of Public Health.

She has published extensively and is particularly noted for her research on Medicaid case management, pharmacoeconomics, and outcomes. She is the only nonphysician principal investigator of the federally funded Patient Outcome Research Teams. She is also author of *The Cost Effectiveness Guidelines for the Evaluation of Pharmaceuticals in Australia*. In 1991, she received the Kershaw Prize for significant contributions to policy research from the Association for Public Policy Analysis and Management, in 1990 the Conrad Elvejam Award from the Wisconsin State Medical Society, and in 1981 the Jay S. Drotman Memorial Award from the American Public Health Association "for challenging public health practice." She is the past chair of the board of the Association of University Programs in Health Administration and sits on the board of directors of the Association for Health Services Research. From 1987 to 1989, she was chair of the Medical Care Section of the American Public Health Association. She has been on nine editorial boards, including all the major health services journals.

JOHN C. GREENE, D.M.D, M.P.H., is Professor and Dean Emeritus at the University of California, San Francisco (UCSF) School of Dentistry. He received his dental degree from the University of Louisville and his public health degree from the University of California, Berkeley. He also holds honorary doctor of science degrees from three universities. Dr. Greene's career in the U.S. Public Health Service spanned three decades. During that time he served in many capacities including Deputy Surgeon General, Chief Dental Officer, and Director of the Bureau of Health Resources Development. He became Dean of the School of Dentistry at UCSF in 1981 and continued in that capacity until his retirement in 1994. His professional interests include epidemiology, disease prevention and health promotion, health professions education, and health policy. He has more than 100 publications on topics such as the epidemiology of periodontal diseases and birth defects and the health effects of the use of smokeless tobacco among professional baseball players. He is a diplomate and past president of the American Board of Dental Public Health. He was a member of the U.S. Preventive Services Task Force and continues on its senior advisory panel. Dr. Greene has received numerous awards and honors. Among them are the Distinguished Service Medal from the Public Health Service, the Award of Merit from the World Dental Federation, and the Outstanding Professional Award from the Pierre Fauchard Academy. He is an elected member of the Institute of Medicine and has served on its governing council. He is past president of both the American and International Associations for Dental Research. He is former chair of the Council of Deans of the American Association of Dental Schools and is a member of the World Health Organization's Expert Advisory Panel on Oral Health. Dr. Greene is now serving as co-chair of the UCSF Chancellor's Task Force on the Impact of Health Care Reform on the Academic Health Center and is associated with the Pew Center for the Health Professions. He also is serving on the National Institutes of Health Advisory Committee on Research on Women's Health and is continuing his work on the use of smokeless tobacco in addition to a variety of other activities at UCSF.

MERWYN R. GREENLICK, Ph.D., is Past Vice-President, Research, of Kaiser Foundation Hospitals; Director of the Kaiser Permanente Center for Health Research from its inception in 1964; and Professor and Chair, Department of Public Health and Preventive Medicine, Oregon Health Sciences University. He is an Adjunct Professor in the Department of Sociology at Portland State University, the School of Public Administration of the University of Southern California, and the University of Hawaii School of Public Health. Dr. Greenlick received his Ph.D. degree in medical care organization from the University of Michigan, specializing in sociology and social psychology. He has served as research advisor to many projects throughout the country and as an advisor to several foreign government research and medical care projects. A major contributor to public policy at the state and national levels, he was recently named Director of the new Oregon Health Policy Institute. Dr. Greenlick was elected to the Institute of Medicine of the National Academy of Sciences in 1971. Dr. Greenlick's research activities have been in the areas of large-scale demonstration projects in the organization and financing of medical care and of behavioral interventions to prevent disease and promote health. He was a co-principal investigator for the Medicare Prospective Payment Demonstration Project ("Medicare Plus") which provided care to more than 7,600 Medicare beneficiaries on a capitation basis. He is currently the principal investigator of the Kaiser Permanente site of the Social HMO project ("Medicare Plus II"), which is investigating the financial feasibility of providing an integrated comprehensive range of acute and long-term care services for the "frail" elderly. He also serves as the chair of the research committee of the national Social HMO Research Consortium. Dr. Greenlick has had extensive experience in clinical trials, both at the local and national levels, and has provided considerable national leadership in this area. He was principal investigator in Portland for the Dietary Intervention Study in Children and is Chair of the National Design and Analysis Committee. He was one of the principal investigators on the clinical trial studying the treatment of systolic hypertension among the elderly. He was also a Portland Project Director for the Multiple Risk Factor Intervention Trial (MRFIT) sponsored by the National Heart, Lung and Blood Institute. He has also developed and directed the highly successful Training Institute in Research Management, a yearly program to train research scientists in managing research projects and organizations. Dr. Greenlick has published extensively in the field of health and health services research. He is the primary author of 41 articles, books, monographs, and chapters and has contributed to 52 other publications. In 1994 the Association for Health Services Research presented Dr. Greenlick its Presidential Award for his contributions to the field.

ADA SUE HINSHAW, Ph.D., R.N. has served as Dean and Professor at the University of Michigan School of Nursing since July 1994. Before that, Dr. Hinshaw was the first permanent director of the National Institute of Nursing Research at the National Institutes of Health. From 1975 to 1987, Dr. Hinshaw served as Director of Research and Professor at the University of Arizona College of Nursing in Tucson, and as Director of Nursing Research at the University Medical Center's Department of Nursing. She has held faculty positions at the University of California, San Francisco, and the University of Kansas.

Throughout her career, Dr. Hinshaw has conducted nursing research, including projects on the quality of patient caregiving and nursing staff turnover. She has given hundreds of presentations, and her findings have been widely published in over 300 journal articles, books, and abstracts. In addition, she has served on numerous scientific advisory committees and task forces, has received many honors, and has been a visiting professor and lecturer at various schools of nursing.

DAVID A. KINDIG, M.D., Ph.D., is Professor of Preventive Medicine and Director of the Wisconsin Network for Health Policy Research (a University-sponsored program to build a Wisconsin health services research community and to conduct policy analysis of state relevance) at the University of Wisconsin–Madison School of Medicine. He served as Vice-Chancellor for Health Sciences at the University from 1980 to 1985. Dr. Kindig was Director of Montefiore Hospital and Medical Center (1976–1980) and Deputy Director of the Bureau of Health Manpower, U.S. Department of Health, Education and Welfare (1974–1976). He is currently Chair of the Federal Council of Graduate Medical Education, and on the Board of Directors of the Association of University Programs in Health Administration and of the Association for Health Services Research. A member of the editorial board of *Medical Care Review* and *Health Affairs,* Dr. Kindig has written extensively on both medical and health policy issues. He received a B.A. degree from Carleton College and M.D. and Ph.D. degrees from the University of Chicago School of Medicine.

KEVIN J. LYONS, PH.D., is Associate Dean in both the College of Allied Health Sciences and the College of Graduate Studies at Thomas Jefferson University. He also directs the Center for Collaborative Research in the College of Allied Health Sciences and oversees nursing and allied health graduate programs. Dr. Lyons holds academic appointments as Associate Professor of Administration in the Department of General Studies and Associate Professor in the Department of Occupational Therapy. He also serves on the faculty at the Graduate School of Education at the University of Pennsylvania. He teaches graduate courses in research design, leadership, and management, and he advises graduate students. Dr. Lyons has presented numerous papers at scientific meetings, particularly in the area of collaborative research, developing faculty scholarship, geriatric rehabilitation, and leadership in nursing and allied health. He has also published in these fields, and he recently received the J. Warren Perry Distinguished Author Award from the Association of Schools of Allied Health Professions. Dr. Lyons has been active in research development on a national level. He serves on peer review panels for the National Institute on Disability and Rehabilitation Research and the Bureau of Health Professions, sat on the steering committee of the Forum on Allied Health Data, and reviews proposals for the American Educational Research Association and the American Evaluation Society Association. He has also been active in the Association of Schools of Allied Health Professions and was recently elected a Fellow in that organization.

ALBERT G. MULLEY, Jr., M.D., is a graduate of Dartmouth College. After receiving degrees in medicine and public policy from Harvard University, he completed his residency training in internal medicine at Massachusetts General

Hospital. He has remained at Harvard, where he is currently Associate Professor of Medicine and Associate Professor of Health Policy, and at Massachusetts General Hospital, where he is Chief of the General Internal Medicine Unit. He is the author and editor of *Primary Care Medicine* and of many articles in the medical and health services research literature. Dr. Mulley's research has included the evaluation of intensive care and the cost-effectiveness of prevention strategies and other common clinical practices. Recent work has focused on the use of decision analysis, outcomes research, and preference assessment methods to distinguish between warranted and unwarranted variations in clinical practices. He recently served on the Institute of Medicine Medicare Quality Assurance Committee and is a member of the Clinical Efficacy Subcommittee of the American College of Physicians.

WILLIAM L. ROPER, M.D., M.P.H., is Senior Vice President and Chief Medical Officer for The Prudential Health Care System, with responsibility for health care operations supporting The Prudential's five regions, and its HMO and point-of-service health plans that are offered in over 40 locations nationwide. Dr. Roper joined The Prudential in 1993 as President of the Prudential Center for Health Care Research. Before coming to The Prudential, Dr. Roper was Director of the Centers for Disease Control and Prevention, from 1990 until 1993. He previously served as deputy assistant to the President for domestic policy and director of the White House Office of Policy Development and was administrator of the Health Care Financing Administration.

DONALD M. STEINWACHS, Ph.D., is Chair and Professor in the Department of Health Policy and Management at the Johns Hopkins University School of Hygiene and Public Health and has joint appointments in the Department of Mental Hygiene, School of Hygiene and Public Health, in the Department of Medicine and the Department of Psychiatry and Behavioral Sciences, School of Medicine, and in the School of Nursing. In addition, Dr. Steinwachs is Director of the Johns Hopkins University Health Services Research and Development Center. His current research includes (1) studies of medical effectiveness and patient outcomes for individuals with specific medical, surgical, and psychiatric conditions; (2) studies of the impact of alternative organizational and financial arrangements on access to care, quality, utilization, and cost; and (3) studies to develop better methods to measure the effectiveness of systems of care, for example, HMOs and other insured populations. He has a particular interest in the role of routine management information systems as sources of data for evaluating the effectiveness and cost of health care. Dr. Steinwachs is also Director of the Johns Hopkins and University of Maryland Center on Organization and Financing of Care to the Severely Mentally Ill. The Center was established in 1987 through support of the National Institute of Mental Health.

The interdisciplinary faculty conducts a range of studies on issues involving policy, organization, and financing of care for individuals with severe and persistent mental illnesses. Dr. Steinwachs is Past President of the Association for Health Services Research and is a member of the Institute of Medicine of the National Academy of Sciences. He serves as a consultant to federal agencies and private foundations and serves on the boards of directors of the Health Outcomes Institute and Mathematica Policy Research.

BAILUS WALKER, Jr., Ph.D., M.P.H., is Professor of Environmental and Occupational Medicine, Associate Director, University Cancer Center, Howard University Medical Center, and the American Public Health Association's Congressional Fellow (1994) in the Office of Congressman Louis Stokes. From 1990 to 1994 he was Dean of Public Health Faculty and Co-director of the Center for Health Policy, University of Oklahoma Health Sciences Center, Oklahoma City. Dr. Walker has served as Commissioner of Public Health for the Commonwealth of Massachusetts and Chairman of the Massachusetts Public Health Council (1983–1987). Earlier (1981–1983) he was State Director of Public Health for Michigan. From 1979 to 1981 he was Director of Occupational Health Standards, Occupational Safety and Health Administration, U.S. Department of Labor. Dr. Walker is Past President of the American Public Health Association and a distinguished Fellow of the Royal Society of Health (London). He was elected to membership in the Institute of Medicine in 1989. Dr. Walker has served on numerous IOM-NAS committees, including the Committee to Study the Future of Public Health in the United States. Dr. Walker is a graduate of the University of Michigan and holds a Ph.D. in environmental and occupational medicine from the University of Minnesota.